Behind the Curtain

Shannon Dingey

Publishing Assistance by
B&T Publishing Services
Knoxville, TN • Nashville, TN

ISBN:979-8-89880165-3-3

Author Photo by Liz Carter
Cover Design and Interior Layout by Tim Marshall
Printed in China

Introduction

Behind the Curtain

Chronic Illnesses are often referred to as invisible illnesses, meaning that in most cases, a person suffering from a chronic illness has no physical attributes that indicate that they are sick. Thus, to the world, they seem like normal healthy individuals. Likewise, because the disease often isn't visible or easily identifiable from a physical or medical perspective, nurses and doctors dismiss the existence of the condition and symptoms.

Having a chronic illness means that the daily battles you face with the disease are primarily behind closed doors. No one sees all that you go through. As if it isn't hard enough enduring the pain and suffering of the disease, you are also in the tireless battle of advocating for treatment and to be seen and understood. You fight the psychological struggle of knowing your symptoms are real and being told by medical professional after medical professional that nothing is wrong and it's all in your head. It's like a curtain separates your reality and what everyone else sees.

Contents

Chapter 1

A Journey Begins

My twin brother and I were born at 32 weeks. Since we were premature, we were in the NICU for six weeks. Shortly after our time in the NICU, I began to break out in hives and sores all over my body. As time went on, the prevalence and severity worsened. After several days, they brought in a specialist team from the local children's hospital and performed a skin biopsy. The biopsy showed that I had a rare skin condition, Cutaneous Mastocytosis. I realize that's a huge word. Well, in actuality, it's two huge words. So, for your sake and mine, let's just refer to Cutaneous Mastocytosis as CM going forward. It's probably not medically correct, but for this book, I think it's perfect.

CM, also known as Urticaria Pigmentosa (again, huge words), is a skin condition characterized by the accumulation of mast cells that present as skin lesions. As a result of this conclusion, they were able to determine that the cause of my hives and sores was the result of an allergic reaction to the alcohol in hand sanitizer used by the care team and my parents when they would hold me. The diagnosis took so long to come to because, at the time, CM had never been diagnosed in a child under the age of two, let alone at birth. Lucky me! Receiving this diagnosis was only the beginning of the medical journey I would face and the medical mystery I was about to endure.

Clinical visits at the local children's hospital and regular doctor's visits were a significant part of my life from birth. Growing up, I had a very different childhood than all of my friends. It began with me seeing a dermatologist every two weeks upon discharge from the NICU. Then once a month. Then, every three months. And then eventually working my way to every six months as the severity of my condition began to improve, and medications began to be effective. The treatment plan they placed me on was an over-the-counter antihistamine once a day once I was old enough to do so. The course of treatment remained the same throughout my whole childhood.

As if this wasn't enough, when I was 10, I began to develop some major stomach issues. I started to get terrible stomach pains and would throw up way more than anyone should. After this occurred for a few months, my primary care doctor referred me to a Gastroenterologist (GI) at my local children's hospital. The GI doctor did some basic lab work and tried a couple of common medications for GI issues, but nothing seemed to make a difference. Over the next five years, I had countless tests performed. There were a ton of ultrasounds and way too many MRIs to keep count of. They tested me for every food allergy that there ever was. Let's be honest; if they could test for it, I was tested. And time after time, test after test, we were left with more questions than answers. Living each day with stomach aches and random episodes of throwing up became a norm for me through my preteen/teen years.

This obviously affected my school and social life. It's hard for me to remember a week that went by when I wasn't pulled out of school for doctor's appointments. I had to avoid certain foods at different times because of the food-elimination diets they were trying on me. These circumstances frustrated me because no one around me had to experience these things, and it wasn't fair. All I wanted was to be a normal kid. And the routine that I was on was far from normal. A meltdown followed most tests because I was just really tired of them. They seemed pointless because we never found anything out, and a solution seemed so far away that I wondered if there would ever be one. I hated taking medication because it seemed pointless and never seemed to do a thing to help the way I was feeling. At times, I lied to my mom that I took my medicine and poured it down the sink instead. Most of the time, she caught me but always met me with grace because she understood how frustrated I was. She would often reiterate that she was ok with me missing a dose here and there but to talk to her about it and not waste the medicine because it wasn't cheap.

Looking back on it now, I question if the symptoms I was experiencing at this time were the onset of Systemic Mastocytosis. I remember a pivotal moment that convinced me this may have been the case. I had a regular GI appointment, and the doctor ordered an ultrasound to see if it would show anything that would determine a direction for treatment. We thought nothing of it because it was common for them to schedule tests before or after my appointment. The doctor called within an hour after we left radiology and asked that we return to the clinic so she could discuss the results with us. Her explanation of the results was confusing, and all we understood was that the ultrasound showed that some of the lymph nodes in my stomach may be enlarged, and she wanted an MRI done. After the MRI, we had to wait a few days for the results. I felt like my entire life was spent waiting for results. And waiting was always the most challenging part. Unfortunately, once again, we hit a dead end. The results showed nothing or at least nothing of concern. However, the enlarged lymph nodes may have been evidence that I had Systemic Mastocytosis or pre-signs of it years before being diagnosed.

In November 2017, the "normal" that I was living became not so normal. For about four days, I was sick with flu-like symptoms, throwing up and lethargic. I could barely get out of bed and was sleeping nonstop. I went to the doctor, and they said I had the flu and it would run its course. Over the next two weeks, I'd find a couple of days where the symptoms lessened, but they were back with a vengeance the following few days. And not a day went by when I wasn't nauseous and very tired. I rarely attended school during this time. Most days, I couldn't even get out of bed. I went back to the doctor, and they reiterated that it was the flu and it would just need to run its course. I was so tired of hearing that it was essentially nothing. I knew it was more, and it was so hard to continue to be dismissed.

I was playing basketball at the time. Well, on days when I could make it to school. I would push myself to get through practices because I loved having that outlet in my life so much. But because I was missing so much school, I also missed so much practice. This cycle went on for three months, resulting in me going to the doctor or ER nearly every week because I was so sick and couldn't keep anything down. There were no answers. Again, they tested me for everything, and nothing came up positive.

Being sick was awful, but at the same time, my world flipped upside down. The life I knew physically, socially, and academically was drastically different than I'd planned. Before things got really bad, I was a straight-A student who never missed school, and now I was missing school every week and fighting to keep up with my schoolwork. I suffered from flu-like symptoms when I went to school because I had no choice. This just wasn't sustainable. I went from being a reasonably healthy teenager to living in survival mode, barely making it through a day of school. Each day I made it to school, all I could think about was getting through the day to get home and go to bed.

On top of being sick all the time and living in survival mode, I lost all of my friends. None of them would text, call, or Snapchat me when I would miss a few days of school. Nor would they ask how I was or if I was okay when I returned to school. They ghosted me, and it felt like I was completely cut out of their lives. They rarely talked to me, and I stopped being invited to things. When I needed my friends and a support system the most I was abandoned. This was the harsh reality that I was living with. I can't say that I blame them. I probably wasn't that much fun to be around because I couldn't eat what they ate and couldn't do many of the things they were doing without getting sick. But still, I just wanted to know someone cared. I missed having friends. We all need people, and I felt that I didn't have any.

I tried to continue playing basketball for a while after I became sick, but I was constantly missing practice. Like most coaches, my coach had a strict attendance policy, and you didn't miss practice. And though my coach was aware of what was going on, my teammates weren't. She kept it private for a bit and didn't share what was going on, but my teammates began to be angry that she allowed me to keep missing practice, so she decided to inform them of my situation so it wouldn't further disrupt the team dynamic. It was mid-December, a month into the season, when I had a meeting with my coach to discuss stepping away because continuing to try to play was hindering my health and probably making my symptoms worse. She agreed and affirmed the necessity to get healthy and keep pushing for a diagnosis. She invited me to join the team even though I wasn't playing. I accepted the offer because I never wanted to abandon my teammates. When my health permitted, I sat on the bench during games, attended practices occasionally, and helped coach the JV players.

To say that this was a challenging season for me would be an understatement. I wasn't Paige Bueckers or anything, but the previous year, I finally began to find my groove and was satisfied with my performance, playing time, and place on the team. And then, just like that, I couldn't play anymore. As much as I wanted to keep playing, I knew it wasn't good for my health, and the inconsistency of my attendance was disrupting the team dynamic, and I didn't want that. The choice to stay a part of the team was a selfless decision. Sitting on the bench was hard. All I wanted was to be on the court with my teammates.

It wasn't only emotionally and mentally difficult being so close to something I loved and not being able to do it, but at the same time, I felt that I began being seen as the sick kid. I mean, I realize that I was sick, but I hated being known as the sick kid. I knew I was the topic of conversation among the coaches and refs before every game. I often felt too weak to stand under the basket or with the team during warm-ups, so I would sit on the bench and watch. I can't remember a game when I didn't overhear the refs ask my coaches why I wasn't playing. When the refs approached me, I felt insecure because they asked, "What's your injury, and how long are you out for?" And I would have to respond, "I'm not injured. I'm sick. I have a chronic illness and will probably be out for the season." It was always awkward because I didn't look sick, and they never knew how to respond. Staying a part of the team and going to games was my attempt to escape the reality of my present circumstances and forget about being sick for a moment. Yet sitting on the sidelines felt like a constant reminder, and it seemed like it was on everyone else's mind when they saw me. The topic of every conversation I had with my teammates' parents after games was my health. I was always asked, "How are you feeling?" or "Will you be playing again soon?" I appreciated everyone's thoughtfulness and concern, but it was exhausting and depressed me.

This insecurity was present in my day-to-day school life as well. The thoughts in my head as I walked through the halls and sat in my classes were, "Does everyone view me as the sick girl?" I wasn't just insecure about the perception others had of me but my appearance as well. I would go to school almost every day with symptoms, specifically bloating, which would leave me feeling very uncomfortable and insecure. I would often have to ask to leave class to take a break because of pain or to go home because I was sick. I learned to fake being well so I wouldn't draw the attention of others and seem different.

The longer I endured this new reality, the more distraught and desperate for answers I became. I was fighting for my life in every sense of the word.

Chapter 2

Diagnosis Day

Finally, after four months of weekly trips to see different doctors and fighting debilitating symptoms, my pediatrician referred me to an Immunologist at Nationwide Children's Hospital (NCH). He had been passive in taking further action, but something was wrong, and we needed to stop waiting and find answers. My symptoms weren't improving; they were getting worse. Even with a referral, getting into Immunology took about a month.

The appointment with the immunologist lasted several hours. Initially, the doctor asked about my symptoms and how long I had experienced them. But after that initial discussion, it seemed her focus quickly shifted to inquiring about my Cutaneous Mastocytosis (CM), which wasn't an issue at the time. She left the room and came back several times, asking about my CM. I would reiterate that I had no problems with it and that the issue was the symptoms of extreme fatigue, consistent upset stomach and bloating, nausea, and frequent unexplainable throwing up. I was frustrated because I felt like I wasn't being heard. But, after about an hour and her third visit, she informed us that she was puzzled about what was going on and that she had sought the opinion of my dermatologist since she had been following my case since birth. She hoped to see if it could be related to my CM or if she had any leads as to what could be going on. Thankfully, the consult was able to happen that day, and finally, we started moving in the direction of finding answers. She explained that there is a disease called Systemic Mastocytosis (another big word that we will refer to as SM), which is a mast cell disease that affects the inside of the body, and they think that is what I am experiencing. The CM I've had since birth could have progressed and transitioned inward, causing the symptoms I was now experiencing. She informed me that Cutaneous is more commonly seen in children, and Systemic is more commonly seen in adults. Being in my teen years, I could be one of the unfortunate "lucky ones" and have developed Systemic as well. She went on to explain that she was going to refer me to Hematology for a second opinion and for a bone marrow biopsy to be done - the only way to diagnose Systemic Mastocytosis.

I left that appointment eager; it was a huge step forward, and we were so close to getting answers. They were able to get me into Hematology within a week. Looking back now, I find it scary how quickly they got me in. The seriousness of the urgent referral to hematology didn't sink in until the day of the appointment.

March 6, 2018

I woke up with anticipation and hoped that the hematologist would agree with the immunologist and they would move forward with the bone marrow biopsy. The car ride to the hospital was like all the other countless trips my mom and I had made. However, the nerves began to set in when we got to the hospital. We parked in the hospital garage instead of the outpatient garage we typically parked in, so it already felt a little more intense and scary. Then, when we got off the elevators on the 11th floor, my eyes went straight to the words "Hematology and Oncology Clinic," and my heart sank and my stomach flopped. The reality of my circumstance felt like I had just walked straight into a glass door. I knew what was happening and where I was heading, but I didn't see the emotions, fear, panic, and thoughts coming, at least not that soon. After we checked in and sat down, my mind was stuck on the question - Do I have cancer? Do they think I have cancer? Why has no one told me if they do?

I never told my mom how I was feeling and what I was questioning because I didn't want to burden her with the thought of something that may not be true. It was like I was trying to protect her even though she was my mom, and she was supposed to protect me. And who am I kidding? She was probably already feeling and questioning the same thing. My emotions were only enhanced by my surroundings. I watched other patients come in; some were happy and excited to play with the toys, and others were very out of it and lethargic because they were exhausted and sick. I scanned the faces of parents and grandparents. You could see that they were anxious and overwhelmed; the weight of the burden they were carrying was physically evident. Then I got called back. A nurse came and did vitals and briefly inquired about what my visit was for. Once she left the room, I conversed with my mom about my hope that the Hematologist would agree with the Immunologist and they would schedule the bone marrow biopsy soon. Then the doctor came in. She communicated that she had read through the notes from my Immunology appointment but wanted to hear from me about what was going on. I explained my symptoms- nausea, vomiting, bloating, fatigue- and how long things had been going on for four months. Based on all the information the doctor and I had provided, she suggested that they would like to do a bone marrow biopsy and that it would be the first step in confirming what was going on; from there, we could proceed with the best treatment plan. She said they would like to schedule it for Thursday (it was Tuesday, so two days away) as long as they could get it on the schedule. They wanted to get the results and start a treatment plan immediately.

I left that appointment full of fear about the what if- cancer. That night, as I lay in bed alone in my thoughts, fears, and anxiety,

I cried out to God, "I know I have been wanting answers, but please don't let it be cancer." I had grown up in church, so I had the knowledge and belief that there was a God, but I never prayed beyond a recited bedtime prayer. I didn't have a relationship with God or know what else to do, so I just cried out to Him. At that moment, I felt God's presence like I never had before, and the spark began my relationship with Jesus.

The next day, my mom got a call that they were able to schedule my bone marrow biopsy for the next day (Thursday). I was glad they could schedule it soon but fearful for the results. However, above anything, I just wanted answers; I was tired of feeling miserable, and no one knew what was happening. Even if it was cancer, knowing something was going to be a relief because at least treatment could begin, and there was a chance I could get better.

That night, I prayed again, but my prayer was a little different. "God, please have the results tomorrow not be cancer, but if they are, help me to get through it. I don't know why I'm going through this. I haven't done anything wrong; if I have, I repent of my sins. Be with me, help me through everything tomorrow, comfort my mom and dad."

March 8, 2018

Today is the day of my bone marrow biopsy.

I woke up nervous, not knowing what to expect from the procedure and with the looming thought of what the results could show. At the same time, I felt relieved knowing that maybe we would finally have a diagnosis. I was silent the entire morning and the whole car ride. There wasn't really anything to say because we were all nervous. My dad joined my mom and me; he usually didn't come to doctor's appointments, but with this being a procedure, he wanted to be there. There was some tension on the drive between my parents as they navigated traffic; the stress of my procedure and the anxiety they both were feeling made them easily provoked to argue. As I listened to them argue, I sat in the back, thinking this was the last thing I needed.

The pre-procedure process was so long. It took a couple of hours as they reviewed my medical history, discussed the procedure, placed an IV, and did a pre-procedure assessment. Then, it was time. The procedure itself was quick, only taking about 15 minutes. I expected to feel pain or discomfort when I woke up, but I wasn't. After fully gaining consciousness, the nurse had me drink juice and eat goldfish to ensure I could tolerate food and liquids before discharge. The nurse explained care instructions for the biopsy wound and that I would likely experience discomfort for a week or two. In all, I was only in post-op for about an hour.

What the nurse said about being sore was true, but I didn't think it would be because I thought I would be fine since I wasn't in pain initially. I guess the numbing medicine took a little while to wear off. I was feeling good, so we stopped for lunch on the way home, and midway through lunch, I began to experience some soreness and discomfort. When I got home from the hospital, both sets of grandparents were there; it felt overwhelming. I'm very introverted, and when I'm in pain, I like isolation and don't like to talk about what is going on. I appreciated their support and helping care for my siblings while I was at the hospital, but I didn't want any social interaction. I made a beeline to my room and stayed there the rest of the night. I was uncomfortable, and my thoughts were consumed by the possibilities of what was next. I wasn't in the mood to filter questions and entertain conversations. Luckily, they only stayed through the evening.

The biopsy was the easy part. The next two weeks were the most difficult as we waited for the biopsy results. The two days leading up to the bone marrow biopsy were the longest and most stressful days I had ever experienced, but they paled in comparison to the two weeks I had to wait for results.

March 20, 2018. Result day.

We had two appointments, one with my hematologist and one with my immunologist, to review the results. The first appointment would be with the hematologist, who would tell us the results. Then, the appointment with the immunologist would be supplemental if needed to discuss treatment plans.

As I woke up that morning, my mom and I barely spoke a word to one another. It was as if we were holding our breath, waiting for the results. We were both eager and terrified because we were finally going to have answers, but it was likely something serious, and it could even be cancer. As we sat in the waiting room, I watched other patients arrive and wondered if this would be my new reality. How would cancer affect my family and my life? How would my friends, teammates, and classmates react? Thankfully, I wasn't left in these thoughts for long as I was quickly called back to a room.

Looking back, had it been cancer, they probably would have called with the results as soon as they received them and brought me in for an appointment or even admission. But being naive and never having been through that process before, we didn't know, and thus our anxiety was high.

The doctor came into the room and cut straight to the results. She explained that I didn't have leukemia, but the biopsy culture showed positive marks for Systemic Mastocytosis. She explained that the condition is rare, there is no cure or set treatment plan for it, and it is treated on a case-by-case basis. There was almost no time to express relief because treatment options were immediately thrown at us.

The options that she laid out were maintenance with antihistamines, which had a minimal risk for side effects, or a TKI drug, which had shown some success with my condition but was more like a chemotherapy drug and had more significant side effects. She further explained that the TKI drug was more commonly used in aggressive cases and those with a high probability of progression.

My mom and I sat there drinking from a fire hose of information, trying to process it all and come to a decision on a treatment plan we thought would be best. My mom looked at me and said, "What do you want to do?" She explained, "You know your symptoms and how you feel." I sat there overwhelmed, having to make this huge life decision. I was grateful that she trusted me and allowed me to make the decision, but I was also terrified to make the wrong choice.

The doctor sat patiently and laid out each option's pros and cons. She validated how heavy and overwhelming deciding this was. She suggested that if I was unsure to try going the anti-histamine route and if it didn't seem to make a difference after a couple of months, we could always reevaluate and explore the TKI drug option. So, I decided to go the route of maintenance with antihistamines. She then explained to me that immunology would manage the antihistamines because they were more specially trained in them than hematology. Had I chosen to go the route of a TKI drug, hematology would have handled that because they were more specially trained with them. The doctor said she was grateful to have played a part in helping me reach a diagnosis, but she was glad that I wouldn't need to see her regularly.

As we were leaving the hematology clinic, we stopped at the receptionist's desk and informed the receptionist that no further appointment was necessary, and his response was, "You are lucky!" Those words would ring bittersweet as I continued through my journey.

We then went to the other side of the hospital for my immunology appointment. At the appointment with my immunologist, she reviewed the biopsy results, diagnosis, treatment options, etc. While repetitive, hearing everything a second time was beneficial because there was so much to take in. My mom and I were concerned about the severity of my condition and whether we were making the right choice by going with the route of antihistamines for maintenance. She explained that SM has tiers- Indolent, Smoldering, Aggressive, and Mast Cell Leukemia (least severe to severe). She stated that according to my results, I had Indolent SM, so it is an excellent choice to start with antihistamines because a TKI drug may not be necessary at my current stage. She then went over the antihistamines she was going to put me on. She stated there would likely be some trial and error as we tried to figure out what would work best for me. I felt more confident in my decision as we left that appointment.

It was evening by the time we left, so my mom called my dad to fill him in on everything when we got to the car. Of course, it ended up being quite a long conversation because he wanted to know all the details. We were parked facing the exterior of the parking garage, and again, I found myself staring out to the streets in my thoughts of relief, fear, optimism, and uncertainty about what the future would hold. I had yet to learn how long the journey would be.

Chapter 3

False Hope

I immediately started the new regime of antihistamines. There wasn't a drastic change. I was switched from Claritin to Zyrtec and put on Zantac. The symptoms I was having didn't improve much. I wasn't expecting an immediate change, but I hoped I would begin to experience relief after a week or two.

A month later, I had a checkback with Immunology. We discussed the concern that not much had changed regarding my symptoms. The doctor explained that medications usually take about a month to get into your system and be effective, so I should start feeling better over the next few weeks.

While the symptoms I was experiencing began to mellow out, they didn't subside. I still struggled with fatigue and stomach symptoms daily. I was making monthly visits to the ER for severe flares. This was exhausting and frustrating because I had high hopes that a diagnosis would mean relief, but it didn't. The only change was that I now had a label for what I was experiencing.

Even though I had a label for it, most doctors and nurses continued to dismiss my pain and the legitimacy of my symptoms. This caused me to question if it was all in my head.

Most of the time, the doctor would walk into my room and say, "I have never heard of Systemic Mastocytosis. I had to research it before coming here to develop a plan." They would then ask, "What have they done in the past?" Sometimes, they would try what was previously done or something similar; sometimes, it would work, and other times it wouldn't. Often, what my body responded to well on the previous visit, it wouldn't respond to the next. This made it incredibly frustrating for me and confusing for the doctors. Most of the time, once I showed signs of improvement, they would discharge me, but then I would get home, and symptoms would come back, or I still wouldn't be able to eat without immediately experiencing a gastrointestinal attack again. The cycle was exhausting.

There were a couple of instances where doctors, in a concealed way, alluded to the concern of lymphoma because of the presence of enlarged lymph nodes on CT scans or ultrasounds. This created unnecessary stress and worry for me and my family as we waited for my care team to look over the radiology reports to determine if there was a concern. Each time, my care team reassured us that the findings were typical for someone with SM. These moments made me angry because I was receiving inadequate treatment and being falsely diagnosed, misguided, and unnecessarily alarmed because doctors were uneducated about my condition.

During this time, I was at a place academically in the second semester of my junior year where I only had to go to school for half a day. I took three classes and then left at lunch. I still had to be full-time since I was only a junior, so I took a college class online that was asynchronous, which allowed me to complete assignments every week and not have to physically or virtually attend a class. This arrangement permitted my body to be under less physical stress because I could go home after school and nap. It also helped me academically because I was missing fewer days of school.

My teachers were very understanding of my situation and would work with me when I did miss school. They gave me grace on completing assignments and would allow me to push back tests until I was ready to take them. When I was out multiple days in a row, they would send assignments home with my mom or my brother, and I would complete them at home in between naps. Sometimes, they wouldn't send home my work because they knew I would do it even if I didn't feel up to it, and they wanted me to focus on getting better so I could return to school. I am incredibly grateful for my teachers because they genuinely cared about me, and their adaptability and understanding helped me maintain my 4.0 GPA despite my circumstances.

However, the decision to only go to school part-time while continuing to battle frequent flares negatively impacted my social life. My distant friendships became non-existent, partly because of my limited presence at school and because none of them ever reached out. Looking back, I could have initiated some conversations more than I did, but I was hurting, coping with a severe illness, and living in survival mode, so reaching out to friends wasn't a top priority. That didn't mean the absence of their presence or concern didn't hurt; it was excruciating. I felt lonely, and it was as though no one cared about me. To top it all off, I wasn't healthy enough to go to my junior prom. My "normal" high school experience was rapidly fading away. And this was hard. This was really hard.

Chapter 4

Silence

In November 2018, my Immunologist referred me to a Mastocytosis Specialist who had recently come to the Immunology clinic at Ohio State University Medical Center (OSUMC). Once I began seeing her, I gained a much greater understanding of Systemic Mastocytosis because she could educate me and provide me with resources that my other doctors had never mentioned and most likely didn't know about themselves. She didn't make any immediate changes to my treatment plan. I began seeing her every four weeks. At my second visit, she upped the dosage of my Zyrtec and added Prilosec as a daily med. She also encouraged me to begin documenting flares and symptoms and keeping a daily food journal of what I ate to see if we could find any correlations. At my third visit, she added two rescue medicines to my regimen: Zofran for nausea and Benadryl, an antihistamine.

Over the next year, I continued to have mild to moderate flares 2-4 times a week and a severe flare about once a month. I was never wholly symptom-free, and it seemed as though symptoms compounded over 4 weeks, likely the result of the aggravation of the mast cells increasing. I charted a flare as any time I experienced a gastrointestinal attack- upset stomach with esophageal/upper right and left quadrant pain. The best way I can describe the pain is a burning and pressure-like pain that feels as though you lit a

5-pound weight on fire and then placed it on my stomach right below my ribs. One of the factors in determining how severe the flare was was the severity of the pain and whether it led to throwing up or not. The second factor was how long the symptoms persisted and whether or not they could be controlled by medication. There was a scale my doctor created to help with the documentation of my symptoms and flares for my doctors.

Mild flares would be when the gastrointestinal attack resolves itself within an hour or two after taking rescue medications. Medium flares would be when the gastrointestinal attack lasts 3-6 hours, symptoms don't resolve right away upon taking rescue medicines, but I don't throw up. Severe flares are when the gastrointestinal attack gets so severe it leads to throwing up, and the pain persists for 10-12 hours, and rescue medications are ineffective. After throwing up, the pain intensifies times five, and usually, once I start throwing up, I can't keep anything down, including meds. During these flares, I would often double over in pain on the bathroom floor, and sometimes, the pain was so intense I felt like I couldn't breathe. Most of the time, I didn't cry when I was in pain; instead, I would go mute and fidget by rocking in a ball, rubbing up and down my arm, or finding a distraction like playing a game on my phone. The result of a severe flare was always an ER visit.

ER trips were a defeating solution now since my Mastocytosis specialist had prescribed rescue medications that were supposed to resolve my symptoms and prevent the escalation to going to the ER. At the same time, the trips to the ER became more manageable because we started going to Nationwide Children's Hospital (NCH) instead of my local ER, and they were more equipped to handle my complex condition. At NCH, the doctors would immediately begin IV Benadryl and Zofran, and that would usually resolve my symptoms. They wouldn't discharge me until my symptoms fully resolved and stayed that way for an hour or two, unlike my local ER, which would release me the moment I showed improvement. This meant a lot of the time, we would spend 12-14 hours in the ER, but it was worth it to have the confidence going home that I had recovered.

I continued to have appointments with my doctors every couple of months and conversations after every ER visit. I had a whole team of doctors- a Mastocytosis Specialist, Immunologist, Dermatologist, Hematologist, and Gastroenterologist, yet none of them could find a resolution for these continued occurrences. Despite nothing new ever showing up, they continued to order tests: upper GI scans, MRIs, CT scans, ultrasounds, and HIDA scans. These tests were repeatedly performed largely because I often experienced upper left and right quadrant pain outside of flares that would persist for a few weeks, go away for a week or two, and then come back. They were worried about the improper function of my liver, spleen, and gallbladder. With organ failure and malfunction being a possible effect of SM, they wanted to ensure they weren't missing anything. I would pray before each test that it would show something. That something would be wrong. I realize that sounds crazy, but I was desperate for answers and something to be treatable. It was determined that the pain I was experiencing was the result of mast cell aggravation and accumulation in those regions of my stomach.

As time passed, it seemed like my doctors weren't doing anything, and to some extent, that was true. While I had doctors, I also didn't because my care was being transferred from NCH to OSUMC/The James, so every couple of months, as referrals were reviewed and appointments became available, I was establishing care with a new doctor in a new department. Each new doctor I saw had to become educated on my case and treatment plan. Much of this came from me explaining the past two years of my health history to them. The initiation for this switch was my care being switched to the Mastocytosis specialist at OSUMC from the Immunologist at NCH. Since she was the primary point of care and

I was 18, it made sense to have all the doctors at the same hospital because it made collaboration and communication between my doctors easier.

I was exhausted, angry, and frustrated during this time. I had suffered for two years with little progress made in the maintenance of my symptoms. I felt as though my doctors were dismissive of my suffering and ignorant of their actions. And while switching my doctors over made sense, it seemed like a step back because it took 6-9 months for my care to be completely transferred, which halted any progression in my treatment. Above everything, I was angry and frustrated with God. Why was I continuing to suffer? Why was I battling symptoms all the time? Why did I have to keep going through tests with no results? Why did all my friends abandon me? Why couldn't I play the sport I loved? When was I going to get better?

Continuing to have symptoms all the time, constantly having to go to appointments for tests, and making constant trips to the ER made meeting my academic goals for senior year challenging. Academically, I was at a place where I could take high school classes or be full-time CCP (College Credit Plus) and take college classes. I weighed the pros and cons of each option and opted to go full-time CCP because although the courses would be more challenging, my schedule would be more flexible, and I would only have to go to school for classes a couple of days a week. I balanced my schedule with two online asynchronous classes and two in-person classes that met on the same days. The in-person classes became more challenging as the fall semester progressed because they had a tighter timeline for assignments, projects, quizzes, and tests than the online classes. Fortunately, I had a 504 plan, essentially a medical IEP, that protected me from repercussions due to the inability to adhere to the attendance policy and allowed me to have extensions on quizzes, tests, papers, and projects upon request. However, I had the same professor for both of my in-person classes, and she was not forgiving and was reluctant to give me extensions and catch me up on material when I missed classes. This made it very difficult, and I often had to involve my disability services representative to get the accommodations I was already approved for. She was reluctant to believe that my symptoms were valid and demanded that I have a doctor's excuse for my absence to be excused or for me to be provided an extension. If it weren't for my rep, I would have failed one of those classes because I had a bad flare and had to miss the day we took the final, and she wasn't going to let me retake it because I had already missed "too many" days of her class. For the spring semester, I switched to the other college my high school was partnered with to take courses, and it worked out much better. I only took one class in person; the rest were online, which helped a ton.

While my academic goals for senior year were met, all my other expectations for senior year were destroyed simply because of my health. My dream of having a senior prom with my friends didn't happen. I was healthy enough to go, but I had no friends to go with. When I tried to make plans with my "friends," they responded that they had already made plans and didn't have room for me. This crushed me. I felt betrayed by my friends and realized that they really didn't forget about me; they just didn't care to be friends anymore. The conversation between me and my friends was very heated and emotional. One of them texted me a couple of weeks before prom and invited me to take pictures with them. She couldn't promise there was space for me to go to dinner with them, but I could at least get photos and hang out with them at prom. I took the offer and was able to find a dress that I really loved. I went in desperation to fit in and not feel left out. I even posted the pictures taken with my friends on Instagram the next day and captioned them: "It was a great night with great people." The smiles in the pictures and the captions were fake. Again, I made a post because everyone else was, but in reality, I was miserable the whole night, feeling like an outcast as no one even acknowledged my presence.

My plans of having a senior basketball season were taken away as well. For most of the summer of 2018, I traveled with my teammates to camps and scrimmages, sitting on the bench, encouraging and supporting them. My hope was by fall, once the season began, I would be able to play, but that proved not to be the case. I was still battling symptoms daily, and as much as I wanted to play, my doctors discouraged it because the physical stress of playing would only exacerbate my symptoms. Not being cleared to play didn't keep me from being there for my teammates. I chose to sit on the bench and support them at every game. My coach was gracious enough to make a place for me even though I couldn't play. She extended an open invitation that, when I felt like it, I was welcome at practice because while I couldn't physically play, my mental knowledge of the game was valuable to my teammates. This wasn't easy. Every practice and every game, I was grieving that I may never get to really compete in basketball again. Again, I constantly fought the insecurity of being the "sick girl." Most coaches knew my status if we had played them the previous year. However, every game, refs still approached me asking what injury I had and how long I was out. I would have to explain that I wasn't out with injury but illness, and trying to explain my condition was very difficult. I was still repeatedly left with insecurity. My insecurity came from my illness being "invisible."

I did get the bittersweet moment of playing in my senior night game, which, believe it or not, caused more hurt than happiness. It caused me to stew on why I didn't fight harder to play the whole season. I wasn't informed that my coach wanted me to dress until I arrived for the game. Anyone who knows me knows I don't take surprises or plan changes well. So, finding out an hour before tip-off that I was dressing made me anxious because I was unprepared. Warming up for the game, I missed most of my shots because I was nervous and overthinking. I hadn't practiced or picked up a ball in a year and a half. It was embarrassing, and I only got more nervous with every shot I missed. My coach gave me the honor of being a starter in the game, and even though it was a special moment, I was grateful to get subbed out after the first possession. Throughout the game, my nerves had a chance to settle. I was subbed back into the game for a few minutes during the last few minutes of the 4th quarter. During those few moments, I felt the most free I had ever felt on the court. I wasn't worried about messing up because there was nothing to lose. It reignited in me a fire for the game that I had lost in comparison, envy, self-criticism, and frustration over my abilities and playing time in the past. At the same time, it was hard to enjoy the moment fully. As I returned to the bench, the crowd was cheering, but the applause didn't feel like it was supposed to. It felt like a sympathy moment, not a career-well-done moment. That being said, I'm thankful I had a thoughtful coach who made space for me amidst my circumstances.

After I graduated, I was still trying to make sense of my illness and how it would affect my future. Amidst the processing of that, I leaned into my faith. I have been a Christian my whole life but never stepped into a relationship with Jesus until my diagnosis. Going through the journey of being diagnosed and then eventually being diagnosed led me to dive deeper into my faith. In the spring of 2019, I began attending Rock City Church with my brother after he was invited by one of his friends. The moment we arrived, I immediately loved it. What I liked most about it was that it was big and no one knew me. We had been attending a church in Mechanicsburg for about three years, for most of which I was sick. I would attend infrequently because I often didn't feel well, but when I would go, it always felt like it was a big deal, and I felt like the center of attention. It just made me uncomfortable. And I hated that. I appreciated the support, but being the center of attention deterred me from wanting to go.

Rock City felt like a fresh start. No one knew what I had been through or what I was going through, and it removed the pressure of pleasing people and allowed me to worship and be receptive to the message. The message the first Sunday we went was exactly what I needed to hear. A woman on staff preached and shared some of her personal story that I really connected with. I felt seen and understood in a way that I never had, and that was the one thing I was searching for at that moment in my life. While her story made me feel deeply seen and understood, God orchestrated it all so that my heart would be opened to him again and reminded that true freedom and complete understanding come through a relationship with him.

That summer, I started reading the bible for the first time in my life. I wasn't sure where to start, so I started with John. I don't know why, but it just felt like a good place to begin. As I read through John, I came to John 9:3, Which reads, "Neither this man nor his parents sinned, but this happened so that the works of God may be displayed in him."

I still remember the moment I sat in my room reading that chapter; when I read that verse, I was overcome with emotion and the presence of God. I felt seen not by people but by God; it was a restoration of hope and confirmation that what I was going through wasn't in vain. There were countless moments when I questioned why me. What did I do wrong? Why do I have to suffer continuously? It didn't miraculously take away my suffering, but reading that verse gave me a new perspective. One I needed heading into the next season of my life.

Chapter 5

Breaking Point

I went off to college in August 2019. I was excited for the next chapter but also nervous about living independently, especially handling my health and flares independently. The first couple of months were great. By God's grace, I didn't have any severe flares. Classes were manageable. I got a job at a daycare just off campus, and I began to make some friends. I spent my nights playing sand volleyball on the court right outside my dorm, which was usually packed with students until 10:30 or 11:00 each night. For the first time in a long time, I felt "normal" again, but this bliss and ease of life didn't last long. As we got further into the semester, the attendance at the volleyball courts and the frequency of people playing began to dwindle because the class load got heavier and we were approaching midterms. This affected my mental health more than I realized at the time; I had become dependent on the relational connection it provided that filled my social cup and distracted me from being in my thoughts. The novelty of college began to wear off.

I chose to have a private room because the thought of navigating the complexities of having a chronic illness and flares with a complete stranger seemed daunting. What would they think? Would they understand? Would they be respectful of my needs and boundaries? Requesting privacy and potentially restricting the roommate's freedom to have friends over and make the space theirs was unrealistic. This decision provided the comfort and security I desired to cope with having an illness, but it presented a lot of isolation from the start. I stepped on campus at ground zero when it came to relationships. If I was going to make friends, I was going to have to be intentional and proactive; this was a seemingly large task since I'm an introvert and have developed significant social anxiety.

On top of that, the balance of work, school, and club activities got more challenging. I was working early mornings, 7a-9a, and some days, 7a-12p, and then going straight to classes. This was hard on my body as I was up late most nights studying, working on assignments, or playing volleyball. I had joined a couple of clubs, CHAARG (a women's athletic club on campus) and CRU (a ministry organization on campus), to make friends, but my involvement in them created a very full schedule on top of work and school.

Cold and flu season hit around midterms. This was when I was the most rundown, and I was being exposed to every virus under the sun. Especially with working at the daycare; since I hadn't worked there before, my immune system wasn't equipped to fight off all the kiddie viruses and illnesses. I contracted a cold from the children and couldn't fight it off. The cold progressed into a sinus infection and double ear infection, yet I refused to take a break from my schedule or go to the doctor because I felt obligated not to miss work or class. Once again, I prioritized living a "normal" life over my health. But it persisted for over a week, so I ended up going to the doctor, and they put me on an antibiotic. The antibiotic they gave me made me sick, so they switched me to another antibiotic, and that antibiotic made me sick as well. The combination of antibiotics and the infections flared up my symptoms of Systemic Mastocytosis. I spoke with my immunologist and GI doctor, who ordered some lab work to see what might happen. The lab work showed that I had developed a C-diff infection because of being switched from antibiotic to antibiotic without finishing the dose. By this point, I couldn't eat anything without going into a flare. My GI doctor put me on another antibiotic for the C-diff infection. I couldn't tolerate that antibiotic either and immediately started throwing it up. It was difficult to decipher at this point if it was the antibiotic, the infection, or the mastocytosis that was making me so sick. We called my GI doctor, who suggested we go to the ER. When the ER doctor saw me, he informed me that I had to be on an antibiotic to cure the C-diff infection; otherwise, it would get worse and cause more issues. So they switched me to another antibiotic but started it as an IV so that it could get in my system and bypass my digestive system in hopes that my body would tolerate it. They admitted me, which gave me another day of antibiotics strictly by IV, and made sure I could continue handling the antibiotic and then be able to switch to taking it by mouth. They also wanted to monitor the SM, get it under control, and ensure they weren't missing anything. I ended up being hospitalized for three days. While I was admitted, they did an endoscopy (this was the first time I had one done) to do some biopsies in my digestive tract to help them better understand the prominence of the SM in my stomach. The results didn't show anything unsuspected; they confirmed that there were a lot of abnormal mast cells in my GI tract. I was discharged with a course of antibiotics to continue taking for a few days.

This hospitalization occurred November 12th- 14th, two weeks before the semester ended. The last thing I needed was the stress of being behind on assignments and missing crucial classes leading up to finals and final projects. I am a perfectionist and a straight-A student, so failing classes wasn't an option in my mind. My professors were somewhat understanding and accommodating; they all gave me an extra week to turn in assignments and final papers, take the final exam, and turn in final projects. I had to defer my English composition class until the spring semester because I had a 10-page paper worth 60% of my grade due as the final exam and wasn't in a good physical or mental head space to complete it. Despite having finished all but one class and getting A's, I did it at the expense of my health. I pushed through for 3 weeks after getting out of the hospital when I should have been resting the most during that time.

Not only did I face finals during this time, but Thanksgiving came as well. Being surrounded by people (even though they were family) and food were the last two things I wanted to face during this time, other than schoolwork. I didn't feel good at all, so no food sounded good, and having pretty much every food in front of me containing gluten or dairy was the last thing I needed to fill my body with. It is most comfortable for me to isolate when I don't feel well, so having to be around family and socialize away from the comfort of my room was irritating and unpleasant. It was more unpleasant having my health and recent hospitalization being the topic of conversation among everyone and with everyone.

After finishing finals and getting through Thanksgiving, I finally had a few weeks to rest. Not much improved. I was very exhausted, and my ability to digest food was poor. Looking back, I realize that on top of everything else, I was struggling with some depression as well. The weight of everything that happened seemed heavy, and I was pretty much spending all day every day in my room lying down or sleeping, partially because I wasn't feeling well but also because I wanted to avoid the thoughts and emotions I was feeling. I felt anxiety about having to go back to campus and resume classes; I wasn't able to recognize that this was how I was feeling at the time or put a label on it. But looking back now, that's what it was.

Then it was Christmas, which was supposed to be the happiest time of the year, but I felt no joy, and my heart was very restless. I was still sick. Once again, I was forced to interact with family when all I wanted was to lay in my bed and isolate myself. Again, each gathering had food I shouldn't have eaten but did anyway, so I didn't have to be an inconvenience. Also, with Christmas approaching, I was only a few weeks away from returning to school. I tried to convince myself I was ready, but as much as I wanted to fake it, I couldn't shake the worry and what-ifs.

Arriving back on campus came with a ton of anxiety. I was concerned about my ability to manage my health by resuming classes and work. However, I continuously shoved the emotions and worry to the side, determined to make it work. But, while I pushed the emotions and feelings away, their physical effects quickly showed. In the course of the last two weeks of January and the first two weeks of February, I made four trips to the ER as a result of not being able to control the symptoms of SM. With each trip, the anxiety I felt increased more and more. As I returned to school, the constant thought was when the next flare would come.

I was back and forth between home and campus, and each return to campus became harder and harder. The first day or two after my mom dropped me off back at campus, I would feel very lonely, sad, and anxious. It got to the point that after I would get dropped off, I would have an anxiety attack within minutes of getting to my room. The last visit to the ER was because I had had a Vasovagal syncope episode at work.

It was a typical work day. I didn't feel any different this morning than I had the mornings before. The class I was assisting in had morning gym time at 8:15. I was walking around the gym watching the kids play, and probably 10-15 minutes in, all of a sudden, I got super lightheaded, and my vision went black, and my heart started pounding out of my chest. Thankfully I was close to a wall and could lean against it to avoid passing out and falling to the ground. I never passed out, but it took me pretty much the rest of our gym time, about half an hour, to feel like I had regained consciousness. I stayed the rest of the 15 minutes of my shift (I didn't want to make a big deal of the situation) and then went straight to my dorm room when I left. When I returned to my dorm room, I immediately called my mom and explained what had happened. She thought I should get checked out, and I suggested just going to NCH and bypassing the on-campus clinic because, with my health history, they wouldn't have been able to treat or diagnose me properly. That's what we did. She left work immediately, came over, picked me up, and went straight to the NCH ER. They did some tests and an EKG and said that it was likely a vasovagal syncope episode because nothing came back abnormal.

This event was the last straw. Before I returned to campus this time, my parents questioned if I should consider taking a leave of absence. Without hesitation, I responded no. I was determined I could do it, and I would make it through. However, after this event, I battled chest pain almost constantly. On the drive over to campus, the chest pain became more intense. My mom questioned multiple times if I was okay and if I would be okay, and I responded yes each time, believing it was true less and less each time, but I felt I had no choice but to make it work and go back to classes. I was so far behind in my classes, and as much as I wanted to avoid resuming life, it just wasn't possible. On the flip side, no one was pressuring me to keep going; the fear of failure in my mind made it a non-negotiable. As I got out of the car, I barely made eye contact with my mom because I was on the verge of tears, and I knew if I held eye contact for more than a second or two, I would lose it, and she would see that I wasn't ok. When I got to my room after my mom dropped me off, I was overcome with an anxiety attack and burst into tears. The chest pain increased, my heart started racing, my body was shaky, and I got a headache. These symptoms lingered for the rest of the night.

I fell on my knees multiple times in prayer, wrestling between whether to continue classes or take a leave of absence. Over the next day, I surrendered to the fact that I was the only one forcing me to stay. I acknowledged that I was a month behind in my classes, and that was nearly an impossible feat for a healthy person, and I was mentally unstable and physically depleted. I knew that if I tried to continue in the current state, I was only moments away from another flare and ER trip that was only going to put me further behind. There was no catching up; I needed to stop everything and heal, which was the reality I had to accept.

I called my mom that evening and told her my conclusion; she agreed and supported the decision. The next day, I contacted the disability services department to meet with someone to talk through my circumstances and begin the leave of absence process. They scheduled a meeting for the following day, and my mom came over to support me. The guy I met with was very understanding of my circumstances and agreed that taking a leave of absence was an intelligent decision academically and for my health. He said something in the meeting that completely shifted my perspective and confirmed that I was making the right decision. He said, "You're not taking a leave of absence because you failed, but you're doing it to prioritize your health and heal."

This was profound. After all, I was clinging so tightly to returning to campus and going to class because I felt like if I "dropped out," I failed and didn't want to fail. Our conversation determined that my leave of absence could be dated back to the beginning of the semester because I had begun missing classes and having ER visits three weeks in. Dating my leave of absence back to the beginning of the semester allowed all my financial aid to be 100% refunded and prevented me from receiving a W on my transcript for any of my classes.

While the leave of absence worked out and didn't present any issues academically, I still struggled with the decision morally and mentally. It was a rock bottom moment for me; yes, battling my health issues was complex and took a lot of things away from me, but now I couldn't even do school. School had been the one remaining thing I could still complete and succeed at. But now, there was nothing to hold on to anymore. College was the path I was supposed to take; what now? Once again, sickness got the victory, and I hated that. When was I going to get the win? Why did everything have to be taken from me?

It wasn't just stress that caused college to become an unsafe environment for me and negatively impacted my physical health. While at school, I struggled to eat healthily. At the time, I was doing my best to avoid gluten and dairy, which was hard when all my meals were coming from the dining hall. Sometimes, I would skip meals because I was tired of eating the same thing, there weren't many options for what I could eat, or I wasn't feeling well, and the food offered didn't sound good or would have only exacerbated my symptoms. When I returned for the spring semester, I decided I would try to meal prep and take my meals since I had a mini fridge in my dorm to store the food and access to a microwave. However, while it was food I could eat, I would get tired of it midweek because it would be the same things over and over. And eating food that had been sitting in the fridge for a week wasn't the healthiest option either.

Additionally, I went to the gym every day and sometimes multiple times a day because working out was one of the few things that enabled the spiraling thoughts in my head to silence for a moment. Working out also allowed me to expend the restless energy stored in my body. Working out raised my heart rate, so it tricked my mind into thinking that my heart racing was normal when I was there. Although working out helped combat the mental stress I was dealing with, it overloaded my body with physical stress because the SM wasn't well controlled. I wasn't eating or sleeping right. So many factors were working against me that I was blind to then.

While I needed to take control of my physical health, I also needed to take control of my mental health. I needed to get help with the anxiety, stress, and PTSD I was experiencing. I had an honest conversation with my doctors explaining that after everything happened in November, I felt like my body never recovered, and symptoms were more consistently present. Then, going back to school, I was anxious about my health because I didn't feel fully recovered. I almost immediately had a flare as I jumped back into school and work, and my body couldn't keep up. It was after that flare I began to experience anxiety about another one because it didn't seem like I could manage them anymore without a trip to the ER, and with that, I was missing more school. I began to feel like I couldn't keep up with school, and I couldn't manage my health. The anxiety, I'm sure, made my symptoms worsen and flares reoccur faster. The anxiety had gotten so bad that I was in a constant attack state until I took a leave of absence. I would like help understanding how to control my anxiety and stress levels so that my symptoms aren't exacerbated by it. My doctor was very understanding and thanked me for being honest and sharing. She put in a referral to a psychologist at NCH.

I was defiant to seek counseling because I didn't want to admit that I was battling anxiety and depression. Part of me was stubborn and wanted to handle things on my own. The other part of me didn't like to acknowledge the fact that there was more of me that was broken and accept the reality that I needed another doctor to help me. Looking back, I question why I wasn't provided a psychologist when I was diagnosed. My doctors had to know that with a chronic illness came a lot of uncertainty and suffering that would likely produce anxiety and depression. Not only was it hard for me to reconcile in my mind, but also spiritually. I was initially hesitant to seek professional help because I believed that seeking professional help meant that I wasn't trusting God enough and my faith was weak. But at this time, Rock City closed a series titled "How to Survive the Winter" with a one-on-one conversation on anxiety with a clinical psychologist. The discussion confirmed that my steps from the leave of absence to seeing a psychologist were justified.

Chapter 6

Breakthrough

Just after moving back home with my leave of absence, around the third week of February, I had an allergic reaction. I tried to eat gluten-free tortillas, and within 30 minutes of consuming my quesadilla, I started throwing up. I could not get the symptoms under control. I was profusely throwing up, and none of my medications were working. I ended up going to the ER. At the ER, they followed the typical protocol for treating me, IV Benadryl and Zofran, and notified the allergist on call at OSUMC to see if they should try anything else. The medicines took the edge off, but I still felt nauseous and still had some stomach pain. They kept me most of the night in the ER since I was slow to come out of the flare. By early morning, my symptoms had mostly subsided, so they felt confident discharging me. They checked with me multiple times to see if I felt well enough to go home, and I said yes, though I still didn't feel quite right. I just assumed I'd feel better if I could go home. We went home; I slept for a few hours but woke up nauseous. I tried to eat and drink a little bit to see if that would help since it had been 12 hours or so since I had last eaten or drank anything, but after a couple of bites, I only felt worse. So my mom called the triage line, and they suggested I come back in. We didn't want to wait around and see if things would improve because we knew we would most likely be looking at at least a 3-4 hour wait in the ER.

We packed a bag with the anticipation that I would probably be getting admitted for at least a night or two. Then, we were headed back to the hospital. And we were right; upon arrival, we had to wait a few hours to be seen. By the time I got into a room, it was late evening. Thankfully, the doctor arrived quickly but didn't have a proposed treatment plan immediately. He didn't want to try IV Benadryl and Zofran again, at least not right away since I had just given it 12 hours prior. He called the allergist at OSUMC again for their opinion on the next course of action. In the meantime, he had me take a Zofran orally and then try chugging down a 16 oz cup of Pedialyte to help with dehydration.

Though I understood the reasoning, it seemed pointless because I knew I wasn't able to tolerate eating or drinking anything. As you can probably imagine, it didn't work. I took a couple of big sips and immediately felt like I was going to throw up. They admitted me after hearing back from allergy and confirming that I couldn't keep liquids down. They admitted me for fluids and 12 hours of NPO to hopefully allow the mast cells to calm down. By the next day, I was able to eat and drink again, but they kept me for a couple of days just to monitor me and do another endoscopy to see if the mast cell presence had changed.

It was after this hospitalization that I became adamant something had to change. I was exhausted, flares were getting more frequent, and nothing was getting better. It had been three years of the same vicious cycle. And now, on top of my physical health, I was battling anxiety and depression that were feeding my symptoms, intensifying them, and causing flares to be more frequent. I hit my breaking point. I felt lonely, tired, angry, and lost. It seemed I would never get out of the perpetual cycle of flares. I began to question if God had a purpose in it all. He felt so distant and silent. I cried to God, "When will the suffering end? "If this is what you have for me, I don't want to do it anymore. I'm done fighting."

It didn't help that during my last hospitalization, the on-floor doctor was dismissive about my symptoms. He kept reverting my concerns to his belief that the symptoms I was experiencing were a result of anxiety and stress, not a condition. For the previous ER visits, that was partially true because the recurrence of flares caused me to develop anxiety as I was trying to manage my symptoms and do school. The present visit was the result of an allergic reaction. I felt like the doctor blamed me for the visit when it wasn't in my control. It angered me.

The following Sunday, the pastor shared a message on healing at my church. This message hit deep because the Pastor talked about how sometimes God does great healing miracles, and other times healing isn't meant to happen this side of heaven. He also noted that it doesn't mean we lack faith if we have prayed for healing and haven't received it. It means that it is not God's will for us to be healed, or at least not yet, and he has a purpose for our suffering on this side of heaven. That Sunday was also baptism Sunday. The Pastor opened things up at the end of the service, inviting anyone who would like to be baptized to exit the auditorium. Especially if you believe in healing to take the invitation of baptism and that you wouldn't just be raised from death to life but would experience healing as well. I was tired of fighting. I was tired of trying to make sense of life with an illness. I was over trying to carry it on my own. I realized at that moment I needed to surrender my circumstances to God fully and believe that He would work in ways only He could. I needed a miracle. I had prayed for healing multiple times along my journey but decided to get baptized that day, believing in a miracle, supernatural breakthrough, or at least the faith to continue to weather the storm. I also believed God would show me the purpose of all my suffering. I wasn't miraculously healed as I was raised from the water, but my faith was renewed. I walked away from that tank believing God had victory over sickness, my sickness. I surrendered my plans, believing that God was writing my story and that whatever was to come was in his hands.

That next week COVID and the shutdown hit. Initially, this met me with a lot of fear and anxiety because I knew my body couldn't handle contracting a virus, especially not after experiencing how the sinus infection wrecked my body only four months prior. This was frustrating because I felt like I was past the anxiety of worrying about having another flare and having to go to the hospital. Still, really, I was only okay as long as there wasn't a threat to my physical health. And COVID was a threat. This felt like a huge step backward. Desperate for change and to do my best to avoid going to the hospital, I began deep diving into research.

I was going to find answers since my doctors couldn't. I gained a lot of knowledge about my condition, which allowed me to be more aware of symptoms and triggers. Through research, I learned that there are different medications- antihistamines, mast cell stabilizers, and leukotriene inhibitors- that are prescribed to treat different symptoms. So, I found the discharge paperwork from my most recent hospital visit to look at my medication list to see what different medicines I was on and what category they fell in. I could suggest changes or additions to my doctors with this information. I realized that I was on a well-rounded regime and couldn't make any suggestions. It was comforting to have confirmation that my doctors were doing all that they could, but it was frustrating because it still wasn't enough to manage my symptoms well. However, through looking over the paperwork, I discovered in my allergy list that I was allergic to Thiamine, which I had seen on the list before but always assumed was a medication since pretty much everything else on the list was, but next to it was B1 in parentheses. This prompted massive research looking up what foods have thiamine in them, and spoiler alert it is in many foods- cereals, pasta, crackers, and chips, just to name a few. As you can imagine, this was eye-opening. While doing this research, it came to my mind to look up what foods were high in histamine, and I discovered that there is an anti-histamine diet. I immediately made drastic changes to my diet, and within a month, I started to feel better. I began to have symptom-free days. I had more energy. The frequent headaches were gone, and I didn't have brain fog anymore (I didn't realize I had this symptom until I began to be able to think and focus better). I had gone weeks without a stomach ache. I felt like I was living for the first time in a long time.

I could also get in to see a psychologist around this time. This was great timing because the uncertainty of whether or not I was immunocompromised and how COVID may affect my body overwhelmed me with fear and anxiety again. I had just begun to feel like the anxiety was gone right before COVID hit. It was also helpful that the psychologist I was assigned to specializes in chronic illness patients. She taught me a lot of skills for pain management and working through anxiety.

During this time, I started running. My symptoms were well managed, and physical activity positively impacted my life. Running became a way for me to shake off anxiety and also a connection point with God. It allowed me to process my thoughts and re-regulate my nervous system.

Although I had made a lot of physical changes, such as diet and counseling, I believe there was spiritual intervention during this time as well. I haven't had a hospitalization since and went over a year after that before I had a severe flare.

Chapter 7

Maintenance

The diet, counseling, and spiritual breakthrough weren't a magic cure for the disease. I'm considered in maintenance now, which means my symptoms are controlled but not absent or cured. My current treatment plan is taking seven antihistamines a day as well as following an antihistamine diet. This regimen is necessary to keep my symptoms at bay and my body from going into anaphylaxis. If I deviate from the diet for even a meal or miss a dose or two of my medication, I experience symptoms right away. The symptoms are mild most of the time but noticeable now that I have a regimen that enables me to go symptom-free the majority of the time. When I felt sick all the time, I didn't notice all the symptoms, but once I felt "healthy, " I was aware of the slight shifts and could better pinpoint the cause. The reactions I usually experience are flushing of my face and skin, congestion, and stomach aches. This can feel defeating and a heavy weight to bear at times because my survival and quality of life are dependent on medication and a strict diet.

I have two ways of looking at it- my freedom is the result of bondage, or my obedience gives way to freedom. And let's be honest, obedience doesn't come without sacrifice. It is difficult and annoying, sometimes even infuriating, to structure my life around my ability to eat safe food and take my medications when I need to.

Being in maintenance also means my life is packed with doctors' appointments and tests. I see my hematologist and immunologist every six months and dermatology and GI once a year. I get blood work done every six months and sometimes more frequently to monitor my tryptase levels and other labs. I have to have regular ultrasounds and scans done to disprove any further progression of the disease.

Also, from time to time, with no identifiable cause, I experience severe flares that result in an Immediate Care Center (ICC) visit. Again, it's frustrating to accept the reality that flares and occasional trips to the ICC could forever be a part of my life. I have found that my anxiety is lessened by accepting this reality instead of fighting against it and thinking I can prevent it. However, this does not make experiencing a flare any easier or less frustrating.

Since May 2021, I have been able to receive immediate treatment for a flare through the Hematology/Oncology Immediate Care Center (ICC). This has been a game-changer for me. When I experience a severe flare and determine that the rescue medications I have at home aren't controlling my symptoms, and I need further medical treatment, I call the on-call nurse line for the hematology/oncology clinic. She puts in a referral for me to the ICC, and most of the time, there is a room available, and they can accommodate me within an hour or two. This makes a huge difference, and I wish I had had this solution years prior. I no longer have to wait hours in the ER to be seen by a doctor and receive care. Now, upon arrival at the ICC, I'm taken to my room and, within 15 or 20 minutes, am seen by a doctor and started on treatment. What's even more amazing is that the doctors are knowledgeable of the disease I have and the treatment plan necessary to control flares. There's no need to explain, and there is no worry that the treatment will be unsuccessful.

Although I receive treatment that resolves the flare, it still takes me 48 to 72 hours after a flare for my symptoms to completely resolve and for me to feel "normal" again. The hardest thing for me to regain is my energy. It gets severely depleted from a flare and from the medication. However, frequently, I will resume life as normal the next day, even if I have been up half the night. It is a coping mechanism for me because I want to avoid dwelling on the fact that I experienced a flare. I don't like to sit in the emotional weight of it. Beyond that, I think it is my defense mechanism not to let others into what I'm going through and be "vulnerable" and "weak." I am still working on opening up and sharing what I'm going through in real time and dealing with my emotions instead of burying them.

Recently, I have found prayer and meditation very effective in combating severe flares. For me, this looks like putting on worship music, sitting with my eyes closed, and focusing on God instead of the pain and nausea I'm experiencing. It is still necessary for me to take rescue medications, but prayer and meditation allow my mind to focus on God instead of being hyper-focused on the pain and symptoms I'm experiencing. Flares seem to resolve quicker now, likely because my symptoms aren't enhanced by fear and anxiety.

Although I have been experiencing flares for six years now and have been in maintenance for three years, flares still haven't gotten easier. Physically, they may be easier to handle for the most part, but they have gotten harder to handle mentally, especially the more spread out the flares get because then they catch me more off guard. Even then, flares are still unpredictable. For instance, in January 2023, I experienced the scariest flare I have ever had. I had a typical mild flare with an upset stomach and mild stomach pain late at night one night. Then, out of nowhere, my heart rate rapidly increased. I felt like I couldn't take deep breaths. I got very hot, and my skin got very flush. The stomach pain I was experiencing intensified. At this point, I took a couple of Benadryl. I was so uncertain about my current state that I texted my mom to come to my room. I wasn't feeling well at all, and something wasn't right. I never did this or even considered it before. It takes a horrible flare for me to wake my mom up in the middle of the night and tell her I'm not feeling well or even express concern. My mom came into my room and sat with me, and thankfully, within 20-30 minutes, the symptoms subsided. It caught me off guard, and it was super scary. We were moments away from administering my Epipen, and the thought of that had never crossed my mind during a flare before. Naturally, I went on a quest to try and figure out the possible cause because if I could understand the cause, then I could prevent it, and then I wouldn't have to worry about that happening again. But the most challenging thing about this all is that there was no cause. The event had me shaken up for a couple of days, but after that, I became at peace that it was just a crazy one-off occurrence and likely wouldn't happen again.

Additionally, being in maintenance hasn't made it easier, but probably even harder, to share the effects of illness on my life with other people. I'm good at communicating what I have been through but terrible at sharing what I'm currently going through. I have some incredible people in my life who have rebuilt my trust and security and enabled me to be vulnerable. However, it's still hard for me to express my diet and needs with old friends, current friends, family, and people I interact with. Every time I experience a flare, especially a major one, I face the psychological dilemma of sharing what I'm going through with those in my close circle, even though they are a fantastic support system for me. I have grown a lot, but I still face physical, physiological, emotional, and social hurdles daily. I still frequently uncover trauma that I didn't know I was still caring.

Chapter 8

Purpose

It was in the summer of 2020 when I had a choice to make. Should I go back to pursue school, or is it best to continue to take some time away? Hitting my lowest point with my health and taking a leave of absence was the reality check I needed to realize how little material and earthly things matter. To realize that I didn't need to follow the traditional cookie-cutter path the world sets out for us. I realized I could make my plans, but God determines what is fulfilled. All through high school, I valued my grades over everything, even my health. When I went off to college, this didn't change. It took being in a constant panic attack state, four ER visits in one month, and being a month behind in all my classes to get me to stop, seek help, and put my health first. But after taking a leave of absence, I shifted all that determination and drive into figuring out how to heal myself and strengthen my relationship with God.

I saw how prioritizing my health opened the door to a "new life" where I was living and not just surviving. Where I was no longer living in the clouds of my disease but seeking ways I could be a beam of light to others with illnesses. My eyes opened to the fact that though my plans were shattered, God's plans weren't. Everything good and important to me was taken away, but what I didn't see was that the best thing and the only thing I needed remained - God. My priorities were restructured - God, health, and school. If school was going to impact my health negatively, I didn't need it. As well, I leaned on the wisdom of God in my decision.

Though I focused on God, I had yet to work through all the anxiety and trauma surrounding my health and school. I felt I wasn't mentally and emotionally ready to return to school. At the same time, I felt the pressure of the world that I needed to return to school because college was the next step I was supposed to take. What would I do with my life if I wasn't pursuing school?

I decided to enroll at OSU, where I could take online classes. I was successful with online college classes in high school, so it seemed doable. Online classes gave me the comfort of being able to stay home- where I could maintain the antihistamine diet and rest around classes and coursework but also acceptance because I wouldn't feel like I was doing nothing with my life. However, school was still synonymous with anxiety in my mind at this time, so I wasn't confident I was ready to step back into it yet, even with the precautions I put in place to protect my physical and mental health.

At the same time, I was working through and contemplating this decision, Rock City Church had opened up an internship program, and I applied. It was a great opportunity to grow my relationship with Jesus and help me discover my purpose. This was God-orchestrated. COVID was still rampant, and colleges and businesses were largely shut down. Which meant there were a lot more online classes available. Having faced the low point that I did and being forced to exit school had me dead set on doing online classes, specifically asynchronous classes, that allowed me to complete work on my schedule. But had it not been for these factors, I wouldn't have considered the internship because it wouldn't have been possible in conjunction with a traditional in-person school schedule. I would have had to choose one or the other. Since I had placed my schooling on such a high pedestal and desired excellence and achievement, I would have never left school for the internship even if I had wanted to because it would have disrupted my reputation. But because of everything, I desperately searched for meaning and purpose. My plans had been thrown out the window, and I felt lost and scared. I needed something fresh and something new.

I got accepted into the internship. But with my overachieving nature and concern for pleasing others and worldly standards, I decided to do school and the internship. This only lasted for a week. After a few days of doing both, I realized that it wouldn't be possible if I wanted to prioritize my health. Although I had only experienced the introductory week of the internship, it was enough of a glimpse to confirm that the experience would be amazing and that it was where God wanted me. I wanted to be all in, not just half in. So, I dropped out of my classes at OSU. I now had the wisdom and discernment to understand my body and mind, what I was capable of, and what was too much, and not to push past my limit. Likewise, I was aware that I was loyal and deterministic. Still, I can't let that cloud my understanding of what would fill my cup and progress my healing and what would drain my cup and potentially derail my healing.

I wasn't sure if I was making the right decision, but I knew I was putting God and my health first, so how could it be wrong? I talked the decision over with my mom, and her response was if it will make you happy and allow you not to be stressed and stay healthy, then I support the decision. Two weeks later, my mom and grandma commented, "You got your smile back" and "You are radiating joy and light and seem so happy." I felt it too. I was enjoying life again. I was in an environment where I felt supported and encouraged in understanding God's purpose for me, and that safety and security gave me the freedom to continue to heal from all the health trauma.

The internship was exactly what I needed; it was a healing experience. I was guided down a path of self-discovery and self-leadership. It enlightened me about how I was created, but it also exposed my insecurities and the things I was still holding on to that prevented me from stepping into the fullness of what God had for me. I was taught that to lead others well, you must first lead yourself well. I had already been brutally taught the lesson that I was going to get nowhere with my future if I didn't prioritize my health in the present. But now I had the tools to take steps forward appropriately. The trajectory of my life shifted. This time, it was in a positive way and not a negative way. I realized God had a purpose for the journey I had been on, and he wanted to use me to minister to people with illnesses and disabilities. I accepted that it was okay that my life didn't look like everyone else's. My view of school shifted. I no longer saw it as a required step I had to complete in life but rather as a tool to fulfill my purpose, and whenever it was part of God's plan for me to complete school, I would. It's wild to think that had I not hit a breaking point with my health where I was forced to take a leave of absence, I likely would have never considered the internship because school would have been too important for me to step away from.

Chapter 9

The "Happiest" Time of the Year

For most, Christmas is the happiest time of the year, but for me, it had become the most dreadful time. Not only Christmas but the whole holiday season, from Thanksgiving to New Year's.

The idea of thankfulness, gratefulness, and celebration felt vindictive. Sickness had taken over and destroyed my life, so to me, there wasn't much to be thankful for. Christmas felt pointless because no gift could excite or distract me from the reality that I was sick and there were no answers or effective treatment methods in sight. There was no gift big enough to overshadow the physical, mental, and emotional pain I was going through. I only wanted to be healthy and have a normal life. New Year's only sparked the grim reflection on a year of pain and suffering, ER visits, doctor appointments, tests, procedures, etc. I was sucked into the depressing shadows of everyone else's highlight reels and celebration of milestones while I was stuck in the same perpetual and vicious cycle of sickness that I felt like I was never going to get out of and I was never going to get anywhere in life. Resolutions seemed pointless because setting goals and dreaming felt like false hope, and I was setting myself up for failure and disappointment because sickness would make them impossible to achieve.

What I didn't realize then was that I had the greatest gift. A gift that takes away all pain and sorrow. That gift is Jesus. My future wasn't empty and hopeless because Jesus is hope, and we are promised that he has a plan and a purpose for our lives.

It wasn't just the nature of the holidays that was challenging for me. Gathering with family during the holidays was very difficult. Two of the most challenging seasons of my life happened during the Holiday season from November to January. November 2017, when I initially became sick, and then in November 2019, when I was hospitalized. From Thanksgiving to Christmas, both these years, I was sick and dealing with a lot of fear and anxiety. Being around family/attending family gatherings was the last thing I wanted to do. When I don't feel good, like many of us, I isolate myself. I don't like talking, social interaction, or others seeing me in pain. As a result, I felt the need to hide that I wasn't feeling well and in pain when I was around family, so I wasn't an inconvenience. When all I wanted to do was lay in my bed and sleep. This made the holidays extremely uncomfortable.

Additionally, my grandparents and other family members would visit me in the hospital, which was unwanted because, again, I get very uncomfortable when people are around when I am sick.

For me, there was a sense of shame associated with being sick. I couldn't accept the "new" me or my new reality. This internal struggle kept me from allowing other people to support me. I didn't want to be sick. I didn't want to need help, so why would I want others to see me sick and help me? I didn't like people seeing a weak and vulnerable side of me. I'm very empathetic. My nature is to care for others to the point of sacrificing my own needs. As a result, people being there for me and sacrificing for me makes me feel bad and sometimes even more anxious. On top of all the internal wrestling, I faced the external reality that the dynamic of all the relationships in my life changed.

Even when it was just me and my mom in the hospital room, I would be silent most of the time because my way of coping is privately and silently dealing with pain. I also need a constant distraction - playing a game on my phone or watching a show or a movie to keep my mind off of the pain and nausea. (The same behavior is true when I battle a flare at home; I retreat to my room alone and distract myself from the pain by playing a game or watching a show on my phone.) I felt terrible to have these distraction methods when family visited because it felt intrusive and unwelcoming to their presence. At the same time, it made hiding and disassociating from the pain more difficult. Having family around during those very vulnerable moments caused me to want to distance myself from them and despise family gatherings, especially Thanksgiving and Christmas dinners, because I subconsciously associated their presence with those traumatic moments. I displaced my trauma onto them.

It didn't help that at these gatherings, I would be asked by everyone how I was doing. It was like my health was the centerpiece of every conversation. Every year, a comment would be made at dinner that it was good to see me feeling better or that my health had improved since the previous year. These moments were well intended but caused a rush of emotions for me of the hard times that I didn't want to experience then.

The association became so severe that every family gathering became dreadful. Out of defense, I would avoid interactions and conversations with family. During my interactions, I would get anxious and immediately begin devising a plan to exit the conversation. I would hide in other rooms because I couldn't leave, but I didn't want to have conversations with anyone. Nearly every time after leaving, I would feel guilty for the way I acted, but my actions were reactionary and not purposeful. It took a couple of years for me to feel comfortable at family gatherings again. It took self-examination and self-awareness of why I was feeling, acting, and responding the way I was when I was around family and then intentionally overcoming and removing the association.

Interactions with family weren't the only thing I had to overcome during the holiday season. I had to fight off the PTSD and fear of sickness. A simple cold or mild flare around that season was a trigger and would bring back memories of the past and initiate fear and anxiety about being severely sick or hospitalized for the holidays. This wasn't easy to retrain; it took having positive experiences during the holiday season to replace the traumatic experiences. For me, this was Christmas Eve and holiday services at church. The excitement and joy of serving others and attending Christmas services enabled me to focus on others instead of myself and the fearful what-ifs that swirled in my mind.

Another thing that helped me overcome PTSD was revealing the thoughts, fears, what-ifs, and internal battles I was facing with people who had become my close circle and whom I trusted. They were able to offer reassurance and remind me of my present reality, that I'm healthy and that the disease is better controlled now. They kept me accountable for proactively resting to combat physical and emotional stress preemptively, thus decreasing the possibility of a flare. They encouraged me to focus on the controllable and not worry about the uncontrollable.

It is disheartening that after overcoming the battle with my health and entering maintenance, I had to fight a second battle, PTSD. There is no magic formula or step-by-step plan for overcoming trauma. While I have overcome a lot of the emotions and reconciled most of the trauma, there are still random situations and experiences that trigger emotions and take me right back. For instance, this past January (2023), a couple of months into starting to write this book, I was struggling with the emotional toll after having a few mild flares over the holiday season due to eating some foods I shouldn't have and getting off track with my medication regimen. I was struggling with the harsh reality that I was still "sick," and without strictly following the anti-histamine diet, I was overcome with symptoms and couldn't function normally.

Until recently, I would have never called what I went through and the emotional and mental battles that have come from it trauma because it seemed insignificant to those who have cancer and other life-threatening diseases. But it was traumatic. I have a condition that has completely changed the trajectory of my life. I have an illness that took things from my life, like sports and getting a college degree. For three years, I lived in survival mode, fighting for my life. I have had to endure countless procedures and tests. Someone else's journey being more traumatic than mine does not mean that my journey wasn't traumatic.

Similarly, I struggled with guilt along my journey. There were times when I had hematology appointments at the James Cancer Hospital or had to go to the ICC, and I would see other patients and feel guilty for being angry or frustrated with my circumstances. My situation seemed inferior to what they were going through, and I thought I should be grateful because my case "wasn't as bad as theirs." Some aspects of their journey were more complex, and some parts of mine were. Their battle was different, not superior.

Chapter 10

Burden

Throughout my journey, I have battled guilt and fear that I was a burden on my family. As I continued to fight frequent flares, I got better and better at hiding when I was sick. I did this because I didn't like attention being on me and felt like a burden to my family. I would fake it until I made it even at home around my parents. Sometimes it was easier this way. If they didn't know I wasn't feeling good, they wouldn't check on me every 15 minutes and ask how I was doing. If they didn't think I was sick, the temperament of the house wouldn't shift. My parents became so hyper-fixated on my health that even a stomach ache or mild flare was a big deal and would change the temperament of the house. It had gotten to the point that whenever I went to the bathroom, I would be asked, "Are you okay?" If I hid the pain, I was the only one that had to bear the burden of it. I would keep medicine in my room so that I could take it when I needed it for a flare, but no one would know, and it wouldn't be made a bigger deal than it needed to be. This wasn't always successful if the flare escalated beyond mild or the medication didn't work, especially if I began throwing up because I could no longer hide that I was experiencing a flare.

I felt terrible for how frequently my mom would have to drop everything and take me to the ER because I was experiencing a severe flare. I felt awful when she would be kept up until late at night, half the night, or all night and would go to work with little sleep or have to find coverage for work because she was caring for me or in the ER with me. I felt terrible that she would have to frequently leave work to take me home from school because I wasn't feeling well. I felt terrible that she was constantly taking work off to take me to doctor's appointments.

As I got older and began to understand finances more, I began to feel bad about the financial burden my illness caused my parents. I began to realize how expensive ER trips were. How expensive tests were. How expensive medication was. And how expensive doctors' appointments were. When I started the anti-histamine diet, I felt bad that my parents were buying all of this costly and unique food just for me. And yes, my parents constantly reassured me that me being healthy was priceless, but I still felt terrible.

Similarly, I felt defeated when I moved back home after taking a leave of absence. I was again solely dependent on my parents financially and for my livelihood. It seemed like I was never going to be healthy enough to start providing for myself and be able to start my own life.

I felt like a burden on my parents because they had to adapt their lives to my needs. They had to bear the emotional and mental weight and stress of having a sick child. Because I saw the heaviness the physical illness caused them, I didn't express the mental battles I was going through. There were many days when I would be having a down day, and rather than communicate that I was sad, frustrated, or overwhelmed, I would just say I was tired to justify why I was isolated and staying in my room all day.

I have never been great at expressing my emotions. I just shove them down until it gets to be too much, and then I have a breakdown. This was frustrating for my mom because I would shove the emotions of doctor appointments, tests, flares, ER visits, missed high school experiences, not having a normal life, etc., down for months and then often randomly break down over something small. Or I would break down after a test or ER visit. These times would confuse my mom because she would try to console me about the event, but that was only the tip of the iceberg of why I felt the way I was. I would dump emotions about several events or things in the past month, and she would ask where this was coming from and why I was just talking about it now.

I felt bad for my siblings - that I was often the primary focus of my parents, taking time and attention away from them. I felt terrible that I was given special treatment or sympathy gifts because my parents felt bad for all that I was going through and were attempting to cheer me up and make me feel better. I got many more yeses from my parents when I asked for things than my siblings did, which has frustrated them. It was never intentional by my parents. They simply felt like they owed me and needed to make up for all the unfairness I endured. My sister has often said things like, "If Shannon asked for that, you would get it for her," or "You like Shannon more than me." Those words hurt my mom because it has never been my mom's intention to show favoritism or to mistreat her, though it comes across that way to her. But I don't know that my mom has taken the opportunity to understand where my sister is coming from and also explain to her the heart behind her actions and saying yes and no.

Similarly, I feel bad that often life was catered to my needs. More often than not, my health and needs took precedence over what my brother and sister needed or wanted to do. Plans shifted or were canceled because I didn't feel good. As we grew up and my diet became more and more restrictive, where we could eat out became more and more limited, so restaurants were always "my" choice. It was the same for dinners at home. Our meals were catered to what I could eat, which meant a lot of the same food over and over, which was annoying for everyone else in my family because they got tired of eating the same thing.

Chapter 11

My Family

While sickness has been a burden for me and greatly affected my life, the effects of sickness have rippled through my family as well. I knew my illness had affected my parents, my brother, and my sister in different ways, but I didn't realize the magnitude to which it had affected them until I sat down and had a conversation with them about it.

CJ (22 years old)

In conversation with my brother, I realized that my illness didn't just cause me to have to grow up fast, but it caused my brother to have to do the same. While the cause was the same, the reasoning was different. I grew up fast as a result of having a disease and having to be aware of allergies, adhere to diets, make major health decisions, and endure countless tests and procedures. He grew up fast as a result of having to step into a parenting role and help care for my sister as I was in and out of the hospital.

My brother felt neglected from time to time because, for our whole lives, I have had the primary focus of my parents due to all my health needs and accommodations. Also, the uncertainty of my health caused the household atmosphere to be troubled and tense at times. He said it was rare to find fun times and anyone to be in positive spirits. My parents were always on edge and prone to arguing with each other. Because of this, my brother sought to be away from home as much as possible. First, this looked like hanging out with his friends and spending the night at their houses a lot. Then he got a girlfriend, and it changed to him being at her house almost every night; he would be there all evening until late at night. My illness didn't just create physical distance between my brother and me. It created physical distance between him and the rest of the family too. None of us ever discussed what was going on, how we felt, or how we were being affected by my illness. We all coped individually and pulled apart from one another instead of leaning into and supporting one another.

My illness didn't have solely a negative impact on my brother. It impacted him in some positive ways too. He said it instilled in him a heart of compassion and selflessness, being sympathetic to the needs of others and putting them before himself. His relationship with God grew, and he sought Him for comfort, peace, and guidance in moments of chaos, negativity, and uncertainty.

Ally (13 years old)

In my conversation with my sister, I realized she was probably most affected. She has only known a childhood where I have been sick. The worst years of my illness were when she was 8-10 years old. She was old enough to comprehend what was going on but too young to know how to communicate how she felt and advocate for what she needed. She was at an age where she was beginning to seek more independence but was still heavily dependent on my mom, so it was hard for her when my mom couldn't be there to meet her needs and comfort her.

The more we talked, the more I realized that my illness didn't just affect her; it actually created trauma. A significant contributor to this trauma was that her life was often abruptly disrupted, going from ordinary to chaotic in an instant because I was experiencing a flare. Although seeing me have a flare and watching me go to the hospital wasn't new to her, it still caused her to be scared and anxious because there was no warning or predictability for the occurrence of one. This resulted in her developing separation anxiety. The majority of the time, my flares would happen at night, and we would leave late into the night to go to the ER. She was always in bed when we left, so she would wake up the following day with us gone and our grandma there to get her ready and take her to school. Even then, she would go to school, not knowing if we would be home and mom would pick her up or if we would end up being in the hospital for a couple of days. If I had a flare earlier in the evening or it escalated quickly, and we would leave before she went to bed, she would often cry, not wanting us to leave.

Additionally, there were times when my mom would have to leave work and take me to the ER. (My mom is a high school secretary at the K-12 school campus my siblings and I attended.) My sister would come down for lunch or after school and be told by the other office staff that my mom had to leave and take me to the doctor, and my grandma would pick her up. My sister would get very upset and anxious whenever a situation was out of her control. Especially if she wasn't provided with the details of what was happening. It created trust issues because people often told her what they thought she needed to hear or what would not worry her. She would find out what was going on later and then be angry because she was misled or forced to sit in anxiety due to the unknown. In addition, she doesn't like being home alone and is clingy to me, my mom, and anyone she gets close to.

Another thing she battles is health anxiety. Watching all that I have been through and experiencing the many times I would go to the hospital has caused her to be fearful and despise going to the doctor. She struggles with anxiety when she has appointments because subconsciously, she is battling the thoughts of what if something is wrong and she is sick. In her mind, the doctor isn't someone you see to stay healthy; it is someone you go to because you are sick. She associates the doctor with pulling her family apart.

Through all the anxiety she has battled, she has learned to cling to Jesus and bring her fears and worries to him in moments of my mom's unexpected absence. She has grown in her faith, trusting God when she can't see the outcome of her present circumstances.

Dad

In my conversation with my dad, he communicated that my illness has had a significant impact on him psychologically and emotionally. It has been challenging for him to watch me endure all that I have had to endure as a result of my illness. The majority of the time, he felt helpless, which is the most unbearable emotion to feel as a parent. He also apologized for being annoying and overbearing during flares when he checked on me constantly. He expressed that it was the only way he felt he could help.

Although it has been unbearable at times for him to watch me battle illness, he said that I have inspired him by my approach to handling it all. My continual pursuit of answers and dedication to researching and learning about my condition has left him in awe. He praised my commitment to a diet and lifestyle that promotes the best outcome for maintaining my symptoms and everyday life. He stated that he knows it is not easy for me to go through each day having to make sacrificial choices and overcoming battles mentally, physically, psychologically, and spiritually. The fact that I kept a positive attitude most of the time has encouraged him. He said he is proud of me for making a life for myself despite my grim circumstances.

My dad also expressed that my faith has inspired him. He has watched the progression of my faith and seen how it has grown over the years through my battle with illness. He sees my faith in how I handle flares. He sees how I lean on my faith amid the uncertainty that my condition brings to my daily life and future and the roller coaster of emotions and thoughts that come with it.

Mom

In the conversation with my mom, she shared what it was like caring for me as a baby and young child - the trials I faced as an infant and toddler that I have no recollection of and the emotions she has felt throughout my whole journey. And what it was like trying to care for a medically complex child while having other children.

Reflecting on my journey, she recalled so many emotions in her mind - terror, uncertainty, helplessness, worry, stress, sleeplessness, guilt, confusion, heartache, and separation. She expressed that her concern and fear over my health have existed since day one because I was a NICU baby, and my condition was present at birth. When I was a baby, it was challenging and scary for my mom. She was a new mom, and my Cutaneous Mastocytosis was very severe. I had open sores all over my body and would cry in discomfort a lot, and there was nothing my parents knew to do or could do to comfort me. I couldn't talk or tell them what was wrong. They couldn't identify what was causing the sores or find any creams or ointments I wasn't allergic to. My parents made frequent trips to our local ER in desperation for help and to soothe the pain and discomfort I was in. Often, the doctors had no idea what Mastocytosis was or how to treat it. This caused my mom to be highly stressed because she had to communicate all my allergies so I wouldn't be given medications or ointments I was allergic to.

Then, when I was two, I started having trouble swallowing, and the doctors figured out that my tonsils were outgrowing my throat. Even though I was having difficulty swallowing and breathing, the doctors refused to operate and take out my tonsils until I was three years old. For six to eight months, I survived on Pediasure because I would choke on anything I would try to eat. Also, during this time, my mom would sleep sitting up every night because holding me upright was the only way I could sleep and not stop breathing. Once I turned three, they began planning the surgery. My parents realized what was a simple and minor procedure for a normal child was going to be a high-risk and major surgery for me. It took multiple consults with different doctors to find one my mom was comfortable with and trusted to do the surgery because the first couple had no regard or consideration for my condition or my allergies and how that would play into surgery. The third surgeon they consulted with thoroughly looked into things and took every precaution he could. He discovered that I had a bleeding disorder and that they would have to take extra precautions to make sure I didn't bleed out. He found that I was allergic to a lot of anesthesia as well. All this information made my mom very nervous, but she was thankful she advocated for me because had she not and one of the other doctors did the surgery, my life would have been put in jeopardy.

It was very challenging for my mom to raise twins and for me to have all of my health issues. She expressed that she is sure that any parents who have a medically complex child feel guilt that their other children don't receive as much love and attention. She shared that I required a lot of her time and that she would often care for me, and my dad or one of my grandmas would be around to care for CJ. She felt guilty that it wasn't often that she could switch between us equally because I had sores or didn't feel well and would require extra attention and care. She recalled a memory of a particular night when we were around ten months old, and I was having a bad night. She was rocking me, and my dad assisted her by getting my mom what she needed. While my parents had their focus on me, my brother just fell asleep on his own in the pack-in-play as if he knew what was going on and that his going to sleep on his own would be a big help to my parents.

Thankfully, as I aged past my toddler years, my Cutaneous Mastocytosis improved, and I no longer had open sores. I could articulate when I didn't feel good and my skin was bothering me. This made it easier for my mom to be there more equally for my brother and me. By the time we were school-age, I was a pretty normal kid. But then I was diagnosed with Systemic Mastocytosis at 16. When I started battling health issues again, especially after developing SM, it was very hard on my mom because my sister was still young. My mom was often torn because my sister wanted her, and she would get upset and angry that she was left in the care of our brother, dad, or grandparents. It was also heartbreaking for my mom to leave late at night to go to the hospital, knowing that my sister was going to be very upset when she woke up in the morning, and she wasn't there. My mom feels terrible that my sister has developed anxiety from those situations.

She expressed that as a mom, your greatest desire is to care for your children, to make them better when they are sick, to fix their problems, and often, when it came to me, she couldn't do that no matter how hard she tried, and that was heart-wrenching. She felt helpless. She recalls watching me throw up over and over and lying on the floor doubled over in pain and not being able to make it better or take the pain away. She grieved with me the missed opportunities throughout high school when I couldn't play basketball anymore, my friends abandoned me, and I had to watch them do things without me. She lamented watching sickness take over my life and keep me from enjoying the everyday things other kids my age were doing and, even more so, stealing my happiness.

Aside from all of the physical and emotional challenges she walked through with me, she, along with my dad, bore a tremendous financial burden with having a sick child. It wasn't something she and my dad shared with anyone. They simply did the best that they could. However, having no financial assistance restricted them from being able to take us on vacations. Mom stated that, in a way, she felt like she failed at giving us the life we deserved. She wished she had documented or shared more of my journey because it could have led to some support. Not only financially but also having a community of people who would step in and help care and provide for our family when needed.

Although my mom bore a lot of the physical and emotional challenges right along with me, the spiritual wrestling she went through was quite possibly more significant. My mom expressed that her faith has been challenged throughout my entire life. She shared that along with being fearful and scared when I was born and immediately presented with health issues, she was angry with God. She couldn't understand why, after going through multiple rounds of IVF and other fertility treatments and receiving the miracle of twins, God would still give her more battles to face. She couldn't get the thought of potentially losing me out of her mind. She wondered, "Why would God take her away after everything I have been through?"

Throughout my infant and toddler years, she prayed continuously for God to make me better, but over and over, there were no answers. She couldn't reconcile why God would put me through all I was going through. And why did she have to continue to endure this suffering alongside me? She would often ask God, "Did I do something wrong? And if I did, then punish me, not her."

As I aged and things got better, her hope was restored, and it seemed like the dark days were behind us. Then, when I started experiencing stomach issues, her heart broke again. She began to cry out again. "Why is she having to endure more? It's not fair." She expressed that the older I got, the harder the weight became for her to bear and the more she struggled with her faith. She was angry with God and couldn't make sense of why I had to endure trial after trial. I would just overcome a battle and be doing well, and there would be hope that things would be better, and then, what seemed like moments later, we were in the pit of the valley again. It wasn't just hard for her to see the physical health challenges increase for me but to watch me face social challenges. It was another heartbreak for her to watch my friendships crumble and my desires for my high school years be crushed. She wrestled with God over why I couldn't seem to have anything I wanted or enjoyed. She begged God to let me be a normal kid.

When I went off to college, there was hope of a new beginning, but once again, it was quickly shattered. The battles and hospitalizations that quickly followed greatly challenged my mom's faith. It seemed like the trials increased each season of my life. She had so many questions. Where was God? Why didn't He hear my prayers? Did He care? What more could He want from me? She felt lost, empty, and hopeless.

It was the worst for my mom when I came home from college after taking a leave of absence. She recalled feeling immense pain and failure as she watched me become more and more depressed and hide out in my room, not wanting to talk or interact with anyone and pushing everyone away. She recently told me, "I didn't know how to help. There was nothing I could say or do." She felt helpless. She would sit with me on my bed, holding me as I cried, and at the same time, she would be distraught and angry about my present situation. She shared that she would sit at lunch and talk with the school guidance counselors, desperate for advice on how to help me keep going. She had gotten to the point where she felt there really was no hope of things getting better.

But one day, by the grace of God, that all changed. She described the breakthrough moment that followed. It was when I got baptized, and she took that opportunity to get rebaptized with me. Watching me dive deep into my faith after that moment provided some peace and rest for her. However, it was later that year, when I started the internship, she saw evidence of a shift. She recalled a few months into the internship, I was "beaming with light." She saw me happier than I had ever been. There was a moment during that season when she went into the bathroom and just fell on her knees. She finally understood the purpose for all the suffering I had been through. She recalled praying, "I don't know why it had to be such a rough road, but I see her purpose and mission now. I see that she is yours. Sorry for doubting you." My deep-rooted faith now gives her the confidence and reassurance that I will not fall into those deep, dark holes again.

Chapter 12

Life's Not Fair

We are constantly inundated with tragic stories of people all around the world. The struggles and trials in our friends' lives, co-workers' lives, and people in our church's lives are always in our faces. We question why so many bad things happen to good people or why there is so much pain all around us. Why do people get cancer? Alzheimer's? Parkinson's? Why do fatal car accidents happen? Why do parents get divorced? Why do natural disasters level towns and cities? Why do athletes have career-ending injuries? Why do people battle addiction?

While it's discouraging to watch so many people experience pain and tragedy, the silver lining is that we can connect with each other through it. This is only possible if we are authentic and vulnerable, share our experiences, and stop pretending our lives are perfect. We often lose the opportunity for connection because we are blinded by comparison.

We scroll through Instagram, Twitter, Facebook, Tiktok and with each swipe, the thoughts grow - I wish I had that, I wish I were there, I wish I had a family like that, I wish I had friends like that, I wish my team were that good, I wish I had that job, I wish I had that house…

We feel lonely, left out, and inferior. So what do we do? We change who we are, what we like, how we act, and what we wear to fit into our environment, continuously changing and shifting until we lose who we are. How can we connect with anyone and find comfort and healing for what we are going through if we are stuck in the land of pretend, disassociating from and refusing to acknowledge that we have a mess in our lives?

We don't just desire what others have, but we also hate the feeling of exclusion, so we overanalyze the lives of our friends and co-workers. We are angered and feel betrayed when we see what they are doing and who they are with and assume that because we aren't with them, they don't like us. This was a consistent theme throughout my entire life.

Reflecting on my life so far, it would be easy to say that it hasn't been fair. I have had health issues since I was born, and a huge part of my life was spent at hospitals. As I got older, I felt embarrassed because I frequently missed school to attend doctor's appointments. It wasn't always that way. When I was young, I looked forward to doctor's appointment days because it meant a solo trip with my mom and lunch and shopping after appointments. But as I got older, I wanted to be at school like a normal kid. My entire life, I have had to take medicine and be hyper-aware of allergies and sensitivities, which made me feel isolated. Again, I just wanted to be a normal kid and not have to take medicine when I woke up every morning and before I went to bed every night. As I got older, I understood that taking medicine kept me healthy, but as a kid, it seemed unfair, restrictive, and annoying. Birthday parties and sleepovers were hard to coordinate, and many times, I wasn't able to go because my health needs made it too challenging. Growing up, I couldn't go to any pool parties because I'm allergic to chlorine. My mom had to accompany me on every field trip to ensure my safety, which felt annoying and restrictive sometimes. Growing up, I was insecure about how my skin looked because it looked different than everyone else's. I was especially insecure when I had rashes, or my skin had flared up. I missed out on a lot of the girly experiences because of my allergy to alcohol. I couldn't share perfumes, lotions, hand sanitizers, or other beauty products with my friends. All those feelings and thoughts were very real for me as a kid but were superficial to what I faced in my junior and senior years of high school.

In my junior and senior years of high school, the most important and best years, I watched my friends and classmates live their best lives while I was at home in bed, fighting for my life. I lived in the shadows of their highlight reels of Friday night football games and post-game hangs at McDonald's, Bdubs, and Roosters. I watched Snapchat stories and scrolled through Instagram posts of my friends hanging out with each other without me. I watched my teammates continue to play the sport they loved while I watched from the sideline, unable to do the same.

While watching my friends enjoy their lives was hard, having a front-row seat to watch my brother (as my twin) live a normal life was crushing. I grew up seeing him live carefree, not worrying about taking medicine or avoiding anything because he had no allergies. He could go to the pool and birthday parties and enjoy everything without restrictions. He could be in other groups and have freedom on school field trips. And then, in high school, he always hung out with his friends, went to football games, and spent the night at his friends' houses. I was watching as he was able to continue to play sports. I watched as he got a job, which I wasn't healthy enough to do. I watched as he got a girlfriend. Even after high school, I have watched my brother's life and future seemingly fall into place. He went to college, got a degree, and graduated college. He's started his career, moved out, and even got married. Meanwhile, my hopes and dreams for my future keep getting shattered left and right, and my status in life remains stagnant. While he was living his best life and seemingly getting everything in his path that he desired, I have had to leave school, have yet to finish college, have yet to step into a career, have yet to be in a relationship, and am still living at home.

We all play the comparison game and feel left out and lonely. But for me, feeling left out was magnified by having an illness. It made me feel like an alien among my peers. And if I didn't feel different, I felt invisible. I sat in tears multiple times a week, crying about feeling left out and wanting to be a normal kid. I felt incredibly insecure because of my illness and blamed it for the reason no one wanted to hang out with me. I was infuriated by the fact that it kept me from attempting to fit in, make plans, and hang out with my friends. Being sick was a piece of my identity I couldn't change or fix.

The insecurity I felt about my illness caused me to develop social anxiety. I have always been an introvert, but having an illness caused me to become hyper-focused on how others could perceive me. Because of the social isolation that I faced in high school, I began to believe the lie that I would never have friends because of my illness. Friendships and relationships were challenging. Starting college, I was still dealing with the ebbs and flows of having an illness and frequently battling symptoms. I didn't know how to share my health issues with others. It's not fun to start a friendship with, "My name is Shannon, I have Systemic Mastocytosis, so I frequently have stomach issues and throw up." But at the same time, I knew that in hanging out with people, at some point, I'd experience symptoms, and it would have to come out. I felt like I was always navigating how to have that conversation. Being real and open about what I was experiencing seemed too vulnerable, but leaving a social setting every time I started not to feel good was even worse. I just knew people would stop wanting to hang out with me. I felt that if I gained more than surface-level friends, I would be a burden to them, and I would hold them back.

The fear and anxiety about meeting friends increased after I had to leave college because I felt like all my friendships were contingent upon my consistent physical presence in their lives. As I was on and off campus dealing with ER visits and hospital stays, the friendships I made vanished. I had made friends through different clubs and activities on campus, but our friendship and connection cut off when I stopped attending because of my health. It was high school all over again. After this, I questioned if I would ever have true friendships that weren't just in my life for a season. I was broken and scarred. I wanted friends that I could confide in and allow into my pain, trauma, and present struggles. I wanted friends that would show up and still be there even when I "disappeared." Eventually, a small group through my church provided this. This happened about a year ago. I had been in a couple of small groups before, and they provided connection, but once the small group ended, most of those friendships ended.

But a year ago, I started attending a small group with some girls I served with in youth ministry. Within a couple of weeks, these girls became some of the deepest relationships that I've ever had. Our lives don't just cross paths once a week. It's much more than that. We are doing life together, walking through the peaks and the valleys with each other. We are all meant for connection, so don't give up on finding your people. You will find them; keep searching, keep stepping out in faith, and most importantly, extend your trust. The love that comes through connection far outweighs the pain of rejection. While we need people in our lives to help us navigate our present challenges, we also need them to challenge us through the fear and paralyzing what-ifs of our future.

My answered prayers for deep friendships have largely satisfied my relational desires; however, I still desire a husband. I have always dreamed of being married and especially having kids. I have yet to be in a relationship. I felt a little left out in high school, never being in a relationship, but it wasn't something I dwelled on a lot. That's not the case anymore as I have gotten older. The insecurity has crept in of whether my health and the uncertainty of it will keep me from ever having a spouse. Will I be too much of a burden? My husband is not just committing to spend his life with me but committing to weather the storms and uncertainties of a chronic illness with me. The fear lies in the fact that that commitment doesn't just come once we are married but comes with the decision to begin dating me. Would any guy be ready for that? Or choose to make that commitment from day one? In sickness and in health. And with me comes a lot of the sickness part.

Beyond the fear and questioning of a future spouse is the fear of whether my illness will affect my ability to have children. The uncertainty of if the illness I have could be passed on to my children. The uncertainty of how pregnancy could flare up the condition. The fear of how the illness would stay managed should I have to go off the medications. I feel like, as people, it's normal that we question our future, and as women, we often question the ability to have children. But when you have a medical condition like mine, there is a whole other level of fear, doubt, and questioning.

With all the comparison and what-ifs comes grief. When I was first diagnosed, I grieved the diagnosis and the present and future effects it would have on my life. At the same time, I grieved the loss of playing sports. What was unfortunate for me at this time in my life was that my grandpa passed away, and my grandmother was grieving the loss of him. Through my pain and grief of battling an illness and her pain and anguish of losing her husband and best friend of over 50 years, we developed a deep and unbreakable bond. There were days we would just cry in each other's arms for hours, unloading all the emotions and pain we were feeling and comforting each other in our incapacity to see the future our lives would hold. I share this to express that in our deep brokenness and hurt; we find healing through confiding in and receiving connection and understanding through someone.

While I have completely grieved the diagnosis and accepted the reality that illness will forever be a part of my life unless God would miraculously heal me, I still grieve having an illness every day. There isn't anything fair about having an illness. There is the burden of having to take medicine every day and organize my life around the need to take it. There is the burden of planning and structuring my schedule to ensure I eat food consistent with my diet so I don't experience a flare. There is the burden of meticulously planning my schedule to ensure I'm getting adequate rest to function optimally and not feel sick all week. There is the unfairness that I have to be mindful of my physical activity so that I'm not causing myself to experience a flare. There is the burden of having to take medicine after I go for a run or play a game of basketball to calm down and re-regulate the mast cells in my body to prevent a flare from happening. There is the burden of doctors' appointments every few months. While I grieve all of these harsh realities daily and how it isn't fair that I have to deal with all of this, I also look at my life, and I'm grateful because despite having to live a life that is calculated, planned, and sometimes restrictive, I can live everyday life. My weekly schedule includes a part-time job, volunteering at my church, hanging out with friends, running and playing basketball, etc. There were days when I was in the thick of my journey when I questioned if I would ever have a normal life again. So I live every day and every moment to the fullest, grateful for everything I get to do and with the perspective that I don't know when something could happen and my life could not be normal again.

My illness has allowed me to be a walking testimony. In sharing with others about my diet, my schedule, etc. I get to share my story, and it's an open door to share the hope of Jesus. My willingness to share my story is an answered prayer because there was a time in my life (as you read in previous chapters) when I hated answering the question, "How are you," and having discussions about my health.

I have become content with my life, where I'm at, and who I am. I see proof that my illness is not a burden but a divine opportunity.

However, I still struggle with moments of comparison, envy, and fear about my future. Still, I know that if you play the comparison game and constantly worry about the what-ifs, you will get stuck in a paralyzing depression that keeps you from even attempting to live life. Yes, feel your feelings and have moments of "it's not fair," but don't stay there. More importantly, stop looking to the left and right and instead look up. You will find contentment when you glorify God amid your circumstances, fall on your knees, and unload your feelings and the heaviness of it all at His feet. The cure for comparison is gratitude. Focus on what you do have and not on what you don't have. God has a great and mighty plan for your life that is unique to you, and only you can fulfill. You don't need what they have. You need what God has for you because what God has for you is better for you than what they have would be for you.

Chapter 13

Show Up

We feel like we have to say something when someone is going through a tragedy or sickness. We have to offer them some type of encouragement, or we have to speak to their suffering. But most of the time, the person who is sick doesn't need to hear a perfectly thought-out speech. They just need someone to be present and listen. It bothered me that everyone spoke at me throughout my journey instead of listening, understanding how I was doing, and simply being present with me. I could hear all the encouraging words in the world, but they made me mad and overwhelmed me because I was consumed with thoughts and emotions I didn't know how to express.

Two phrases I grew to despise throughout my journey were "How are you?" and "It will be ok."

Most of us ask the question "How are you?" in passing and in an ingenious way. How often do we take the time to listen to the person's response? I feel like, in most cases, we just ask it out of default because it is a question we are supposed to ask. We are all guilty of asking a person how they are and then continuing to do whatever we are doing before they even respond because we expect them just to say I'm good, and that's it. When I was sick, I was asked, "How are you?" I often responded, "I'm good," because I didn't want to burden the other person, and I honestly wasn't sure they cared to know how I really was. I didn't want them to carry my burden.

"How are you?" became a triggering phrase for me to answer. If I responded genuinely, then I had to be vulnerable, which I hated, but if I responded, "I'm good," then I felt I was blatantly lying to the person's face. Most of the time, I didn't feel like answering many follow-up questions either, so responding "I'm good" was my best shot at dodging any further conversation. Yet, every conversation was a reminder of my health.

Additionally, to maintain a sense of normalcy and privacy, I was always hyper-aware that no one saw that I wasn't ok. Expressing that I wasn't okay in conversation or by how I presented myself was usually followed by a sympathetic or encouraging speech of I'm sorry, and I hope things get better soon. This caused me to begin to avoid conversations with everyone. I wanted to feel seen and supported. I wanted outlets to share what was happening and, most importantly, how I felt. But most people just couldn't understand it. It's not their fault; I just didn't want to have to explain why I wasn't okay all the time.

I had similar feelings about the phrase "It will be ok." Too often, I was met with one-sided conversations of someone encouraging me that everything would be ok without taking the time to hear and understand how I felt. This especially felt insensitive when I was in the hospital recovering from a flare when everyone around me would tell me everything would be okay. For me, nothing about my situation felt okay. While I was getting better, I knew another flare was around the corner. I didn't know when we would have answers and a treatment plan that worked to combat the debilitating symptoms I continued to experience daily. I felt the same way when I would have procedures done. I was told before going in that, "Everything will be ok." I wasn't concerned about the procedure or the recovery. My concern and distress lay in questioning whether the test results would show anything or if they would return as nothing again. With each procedure and test, my confidence in the results identifying something treatable or providing answers or direction for treatment dwindled and thus made the phrase, "everything will be ok," more infuriating. My situation wasn't okay. I was enduring yet another painful, stressful, and pointless procedure for nothing to come from it. It was less about the present event and more about my overall circumstances and how I felt. Nothing about my life felt okay - my symptoms weren't getting any better, there were no answers in sight, my friends vanished, I couldn't play basketball, I was pouring everything I had into keeping up with school, and I was battling anxiety. Everything was uncertain, confusing, and exhausting. Being told repeatedly that everything would be okay made me feel like I had to be okay. I needed a shoulder, not a sermon. I wanted someone to be present and just sit with me and let me cry and be "weak" and not have it all together for a moment. Someone to hear me out, let me express my emotions, and take time to understand how I felt.

Even amid all the pain and suffering, I was going through, I still felt the need to please other people - not to inconvenience them or hurt their feelings - even though it often meant compromising my own needs, wants, and comfort. Let me encourage you to be selfish if you are facing a health battle or something similar. Ask for privacy when you need it, refuse visitors when you need to, ask people to be quiet and just listen or be present when you need to, cry when you need to, and vent when you need to. Don't hide and conceal your emotions and desires. What is best for you is what is most important. At the same time, let your people in. They can't help you if they don't know what you need or when and how you struggle. Your community can't show up for you if you shut them out.

If you are supporting someone battling illness or grieving a tragedy, the best question you can ask is, "What do you need?" That question puts the control in their hands. It allows them to communicate their emotions and desires. It enables them to say I need to be alone. I just need someone to listen. I need to talk. I need to cry. I need to vent. I need you to make me laugh or cheer me up. I need to go somewhere or do something. I just want someone to be present with me, etc. If they don't know what they need, just show up, and be present. Sometimes they don't know what they need. So just show up and love them.

Another tip for those supporting someone battling illness is to take a step back and reflect on their type of person and how they cope. Do they like interaction when they are sick, or do they like solitude? Do they openly share what they are going through and initiate conversation, or do they need space or a push to open up? Do you know their cues when they are stressed or struggling? Knowing and being observant about these things will help you serve the other person well and help them feel seen and cared for.

Chapter 14

Faith

When it comes to battling a chronic illness, a disease, or a disability, faith can be a topic of tension. Maybe you grew up believing in God, but then you had a child with a disability or your child was diagnosed with an illness, and you walked away from your faith. Maybe you were rejected by the church because your child has a disability. Maybe you grew up in a religious family, and you got sick, and all your family and church have done is dismiss your symptoms and suffering instead of walking alongside you through it. Maybe you're ill, and you are wrestling between trusting God and seeking medical intervention. Maybe you are facing a crisis of faith because you are still waiting for your miracle or breakthrough. Maybe you believe and trust God, but he didn't answer your prayers as you thought he would.

I have had multiple crises of faith moments throughout my health journey. I have hit the crossroads of believing that God is good, works everything for his good, and has a plan despite having no sight of a breakthrough and throwing it all away.

A moment of crisis of faith initiated my relationship with Jesus. If I hadn't developed Systemic Mastocytosis, needed a bone marrow biopsy, and had the fear that I may have cancer, I may have never pursued a relationship with Jesus. Had I not had two hospitalizations and hit rock bottom physically and mentally in February 2020 and chose to cling to Jesus despite all the uncertainty then and through COVID, I wouldn't have stepped away from school and pursued the internship. The internship helped me discover my purpose and encouraged me to share my story; it birthed a passion inside of me that led to writing this book. In those two defining moments, I had to choose who or what I would put my faith and hope in.

Though I chose Jesus in those moments, I have wrestled through my whole journey with why I continued to suffer if God is good. I fought debilitating symptoms for three years with no answers or stabilization. I had all my hopes for the present and future taken from me. While it is easy to blame God and righteous to question why, God didn't take basketball, school, and my plans for the future away from me; sickness did. God allowed all of those events to play out so that His greater plan could be carried out. He wasn't silent or absent through my suffering. Even though it seemed that way, He was merciful. He could have shortened my desert season, but what greater story has He written through my suffering?

Similarly, I have the unique circumstance that a gene mutation causes Systemic Mastocytosis. I have to believe that God wrote SM in His plan for me if I believe the verse, "He knit me together in my mother's womb, and I am fearfully and wonderfully made." It is hard to believe that God, who created the whole earth perfectly, would make a mistake in creating me. I know that for many who suffer from a chronic illness, there is no explanation for their suffering. There is nothing it can be linked or traced to, which leaves a huge gap for questioning the purpose behind the pain. If you are suffering from a chronic illness, you have likely been blamed for your suffering - "You didn't take care of yourself," "It's all in your head," or "You're too stressed." But John 9:3 says, "Neither this man nor his parents sinned, but this happened so that the works of God may be displayed in Him." Your illness is not your fault. This verse says that God is allowing you to experience what you are going through because it is part of His plan to bring others to know him. If you are anything like me, this is extremely difficult to reconcile; there have been more times than I can count that I have cried out to God with transparency, "I don't want to do this anymore, I can't do this anymore if this is the path you have for me I don't want it." These are crisis of faith moments where we can either surrender to God and trust that He will carry us through, or we throw in the towel and walk away from our faith. The battle may not get easier, but I know there will be purpose in the pain if I place my faith in God. The fight becomes much easier when I rely on God's strength, not my own, to carry me through. We don't battle suffering and pain because we deserve it. We battle suffering and pain because God has chosen to use us.

You may still be questioning why I or anyone else must battle sickness. The answer is that sickness entered the world as a result of sin. When humans chose to eat the fruit in the garden, we invited sin, sickness, pain, and suffering into the world. We enabled sickness to run rampant through our world, not God. You may ask, how is God good and all-powerful if He can't rid the world of sickness? He can. We hear of miracles every day of God's healing power. We also hear every day of people being given devastating and terminal diagnoses. But God is still God in both scenarios. He uses both for his glory. Have you ever followed someone's story that has faced a terminal illness or injury and not been inspired or changed? Conversely, it's okay to ask the big questions or to wrestle with God. To search for the truth and run to the one who is the truth.

Living with a chronic illness is moment by moment surrender to God. In the valleys of my journey, I had to surrender to God because I couldn't make it through otherwise. Now, I surrender the fear of a flare when I begin to experience symptoms. I surrender the fear and question about my future. I surrender the authority and power sickness tries to have over my life.

Surrender also looks like not letting our diagnosis or circumstance be a god in our life. I struggled with SM being "god" in my life. I let the past, present, and future effects of it rule my life. I let it dictate how I lived my life instead of living in a way that supported my health. I have lived in fear and anxiety of a flare. In surrendering my illness to God, disease no longer has authority over my life. I began to view my circumstances from a heavenly perspective, not an earthly one. I no longer fear the possibility of flares because I know that He will bring me through. I no longer fear or worry about my future because I know that whatever God has planned is bigger than anything I could dream of. I no longer try to control what is uncontrollable but recognize that even though sickness is out of my control, it isn't out of God's control.

Similarly, I allowed sickness to become the strongest piece of my identity. Once I was healthy enough to live a normal life, I still lived like I was sick because that was what I knew and what felt comfortable. Sickness hadn't just gained power over my life but also who I was. I struggled greatly with how others saw me because I saw myself as sick. Sickness distorted how I saw my future and what I thought I could accomplish. But while I saw myself as sick, God saw me as healed and purposed.

Additionally, throughout my journey, the thing I desired most besides being healed was someone or a group of people who understood what I was going through and how I felt. Not just someone who could sympathize with me but someone who could empathize with me. I am still looking for that. I have yet to meet someone who has the condition I have and understands what I have been through. But even if I meet someone with SM who can understand what it is like to battle it, our experiences wouldn't be the same. God is the only person who completely understands what I'm going through. The one who created me. The one who experienced and conquered all things and did the impossible, rising from death to life.

Postlude

Dear Me

Dear 16-year-old me (the one who was recently diagnosed with illness),

Your world seems so dark and scary right now. You are frustrated, angry, confused, worried, and exhausted. Your life seems so unfair. You felt fine, and then suddenly, you were super sick. You have been fighting for answers for months, and now you finally have answers, but the path forward is still very unclear. You are relieved to have a diagnosis but scared of what the future holds and if you are making the right decisions when it comes to treatment options. You are coming to terms with the reality that you can't play sports now; you were a healthy teenager, and then in a blink, you can barely get out of bed. You are not only feeling the physical and mental pain of having an illness and making sense of a new diagnosis, but you are bearing the emotional pain of friendships in your life changing and becoming nonexistent. It seems as though everything you have wanted for your high school career is slipping away. In the midst of all of this, though, you have found the greatest thing, and that is God. Lean into your relationship with Him, and keep pursuing Him no matter how long and hard the journey gets. The journey is going to be long, and it is going to get darker, but there is light, and you will see that there is purpose for everything you are going through and will go through. Don't lose hope. Don't ever lose hope.

I know you are a people pleaser and don't like attention, but lean into the support system that you have. Express your emotions, your needs, and your wants even though you don't want to because it will bring relief and make things easier for you. It isn't your job to bear the weight alone or be uncomfortable so that others aren't burdened. Let them take the weight, don't fear their response or hold yourself responsible for their reactions to your wishes. At the same time, despite your insecurity, let people help you, check on you, and care for you. Don't stop advocating for yourself. You are going to continue to face doctors who don't know how to treat you, what your condition is, and who will dismiss your symptoms. What you are experiencing is real, and your symptoms are real. Don't believe the lies of doctors or nurses or even yourself that say that it is all in your head. You're making yourself sick, or you're exaggerating. Document your journey, journal your thoughts, and your emotions. Not only will it help you cope now, but it will be encouraging to look back on later. Take pictures and videos. They will help you remember how far you've come.

Dear 18-year-old self,

You feel physically, emotionally, mentally, and spiritually defeated. You're discouraged and exhausted. It seems as though everything you wanted for your future is slipping through your fingers. You have been fighting for two years, and things seem to worsen. You are frustrated that your health is diminishing your quality of life and vision for your future. Your hopes of stepping out and starting your own life have been crushed. You're at a loss for where to go from here. Your only focus right now should be your health and taking time to heal. It is frustrating that you have to pause your life to focus on your health, but your dreams and plans are never going to be possible if your health is not stabilized. You have pushed through and pushed through, striving to keep your life moving forward, but taking a break is ok - press pause. Life will be there when you are physically and mentally healthy enough to continue. Don't lose hope. Things will get better. I know it seems like the suffering is never going to end. It seems like doctors aren't hearing you, believing you, or taking your pain and symptoms seriously. It seems like they are never going to find answers. It feels like the days are getting darker. You're desperate for answers for something to work. Hang on, there will be a breakthrough. You are going to realize your purpose and calling through this journey. You will look back on this time as one of the most influential times in your life when your priorities shifted, and the tide turned.

Epilogue

To the Ones Who Know Me Best and Love Me Most

Dear Siblings,

You are not forgotten. I see you. I apologize, on behalf of your circumstance, that you don't receive as much time and attention as your medically complex sibling. I'm sorry that you had to grow up and become independent faster because you had to meet your needs when your mom and dad were preoccupied. I'm sorry you have had to make many sacrifices and have had your preferences overridden repeatedly. I'm sorry that I have stolen experiences from you. I (on behalf of the medically complex child) feel bad for the burden and stress I have caused in your life and the time and attention I have taken away from you. Thank you for continuing to show up and care for me even when you probably didn't want to and were frustrated by how the present circumstances were affecting your life. Thank you for comforting me and encouraging me when I need it.

At the same time, I want you to know your feelings, thoughts, and emotions are valid. Don't hold them in. Share them with Mom and Dad. Share them with me. I won't be offended. I promise. I want to be there for you and support you just like you are there for me. Feeling forgotten, neglected, annoyed, frustrated, and angry is normal. Your challenges and difficulties in life are not less than they are different. Though it has been a challenge and, most of the time, not easy, your experiences have shaped you greatly, some negatively, but mostly positively. You are more empathetic, observant, selfless, and compassionate because you have had to look after and grow up with me. You have a positive outlook because you understand life's short and uncertainness. God chose you to be the sibling of a child with an illness/disability because the experience will aid in shaping and molding you into who He created you to be and lead you to the calling He has for you.

Dear Parents,

I don't think there are words to express my gratitude for your love and care through my journey so far and your continued love and support. You have endured countless sleepless nights caring for and worrying about me. Your sacrifice in laying down your life and preferences so that I am cared for, and my needs are met. Your commitment to advocating for me when doctors wouldn't listen or weren't concerned enough. Your devotion to caring for me daily. Your grace and compassion when I would get angry and frustrated about my circumstances, taking medication, and not being a normal kid. Your listening ear when I need space to scream and cry.

Your sacrifice and the stress you endured financially to make sure I received the care and medication I needed when I needed it. I can only see my fight and my journey from my perspective. I can't fully comprehend the effect it has had and continues to have on you.

Yes, I have endured firsthand the pain and suffering that comes with battling an incurable illness, but you have had to watch your child endure pain and suffering that you aren't able to take away.

Just like I have questioned, why me? What did I do to deserve this? I'm sure you have asked similar questions.

But though it may seem like a punishment, I believe it is a blessing. I believe God saw something in you that set you apart and made you worthy to be given the gift of raising a child with an illness/disability. However, saying you should see it as a blessing doesn't mean you should feel guilty for any negative emotions you feel. All of those are valid. The feeling of inadequacy to bear the burden, to provide the support and care needed, and to find a solution. The physical, emotional, and psychological pain of watching your child suffer. The frustration with the doctors for not listening and not finding answers, and with the reality that there aren't answers. The stress of balancing work, life, parenting, and finances to seek the best treatment for your child possible - to see the best doctors, to travel to the best facilities, to do the trials that offer a cure or longer life, to do the procedures that could lead to answers, to purchase the medication that isn't covered by insurance but offers relief and control of symptoms, etc. The heartache of letting down your other children and the inability to equally care for and support them. The distress in the fight to keep your marriage alive as you are exhausted and wounded from caring for a medically complex child.

When you feel these emotions, and like you're at the end, and it is too much to bear, you should fall on your knees, cry out to God, and let Him carry the burden and weight. You don't have to and aren't supposed to walk through it alone.